Carcinoma of the Bladder

Edited by

David MacVicar

Series Editor

Rodney H. Reznek

Editorial Adviser

Janet E. Husband

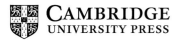

CAMBRIDGE
UNIVERSITY PRESS

CAMBRIDGE UNIVERSITY PRESS
Cambridge, New York, Melbourne, Madrid, Cape Town, Singapore, São Paulo, Delhi

Cambridge University Press
The Edinburgh Building, Cambridge CB2 8RU, UK

Published in the United States of America by Cambridge University Press, New York

www.cambridge.org
Information on this title: www.cambridge.org/9780521884563

First published 2008

Printed in the United Kingdom at the University Press, Cambridge

A catalog record for this publication is available from the British Library

Library of Congress Cataloging in Publication data
Carcinoma of the bladder / edited by David MacVicar.
    p.   ;   cm. — (Contemporary issues in cancer imaging)
Includes bibliographical references and index.
ISBN 978-0-521-88456-3 (hardback)
I. MacVicar, David.   II. Series.
[DNLM: 1. Urinary Bladder Neoplasms—radiography.   2. Urinary Bladder Neoplasms—therapy.
WJ 504 C2651 2008]
RC280.B5C3413 2008
616.99′462—dc22
                                                                                2007048758
ISBN 978-0-521-88456-3 hardback

Contents

Color plates are situated between pages 20 and 21

Contributors

Jonathan Berry
Consultant Radiologist
Department of Diagnostic Radiology
Cumberland Infirmary
Carlisle, UK

Suzanne Bonington
Consultant Radiologist
Department of Diagnostic Radiology
Christie Hospital
Manchester, UK

Bernadette Carrington
Consultant Radiologist
Department of Diagnostic Radiology
Christie Hospital
Manchester, UK

Robert Huddart
Senior Lecturer & Honorary Consultant in
Clinical Oncology & Radiotherapy
Department of Radiotherapy
Royal Marsden Hospital
Sutton, UK

Charles Jameson
Consultant Histopathologist
Histopathology Department
Royal Marsden Hospital
London, UK

Susan Lalondrelle
Research Fellow
Department of Radiotherapy
Royal Marsden Hospital
Sutton, UK

David MacVicar
Consultant Radiologist
Department of Diagnostic Radiology
Royal Marsden Hospital
Sutton, UK

Delia Pudney
Specialist Registrar
Department of Radiotherapy
Royal Marsden Hospital
Sutton, UK

Sarb Sandhu
Locum Consultant Urologist
Urology Unit
Royal Marsden Hospital
London, UK

Aslam Sohaib
Consultant Radiologist
Department of Diagnostic Radiology
Royal Marsden Hospital
London, UK

Joanne Stokoe
Specialist Registrar
Department of Radiotherapy
Royal Marsden Hospital
Sutton, UK

Ben Taylor
Consultant Radiologist
Department of Diagnostic Radiology
Christie Hospital
Manchester, UK

Alan Thompson
Consultant Urologist Surgeon
Urology Unit
Royal Marsden Hospital
London, UK

Camilla Whitten
Specialist Registrar
Department of Diagnostic Radiology
Royal Marsden Hospital
Sutton, UK

Sarah Williams
Specialist Registrar
Department of Diagnostic Radiology
Royal Marsden Hospital
Sutton, UK

Series foreword

Imaging has become pivotal in all aspects of the management of patients with cancer. At the same time it is acknowledged that optimal patient care is best achieved by a multidisciplinary team approach. The explosion of technological developments in imaging over the past years has meant that all members of the multidisciplinary team should understand the potential applications, limitations and advantages of all the evolving and exciting imaging techniques. Equally, to understand the significance of the imaging findings and to contribute actively to management decisions and to the development of new clinical applications for imaging, it is critical that the radiologist should have sufficient background knowledge of different tumors. Thus the radiologist should understand the pathology, the clinical background, the therapeutic options and prognostic indicators of malignancy.

Contemporary Issues in Cancer Imaging – A Multidisciplinary Approach aims to meet the growing requirement for radiologists to have detailed knowledge of the individual tumors in which they are involved in making management decisions. A series of single subject issues, each of which will be dedicated to a single tumor site, edited by recognised expert guest editors, will include contributions from basic scientists, pathologists, surgeons, oncologists, radiologists and others.

While the series is written predominantly for the radiologist, it is hoped that individual issues will contain sufficient varied information so as to be of interest to all medical disciplines and to other health professionals managing patients with cancer. As with imaging, advances have occurred in all these disciplines related to cancer management and it is our fervent hope that this series, bringing together expertise from such a range of related specialties, will not only promote the understanding and rational application of modern imaging but will also help to achieve the ultimate goal of improving outcomes for patients with cancer.

Rodney H. Reznek
London

Preface to Carcinoma of the Bladder

Cancer of the urinary bladder encompasses a range of cell types, the most common in Western societies being transitional cell carcinoma (TCC). These neoplasms are characterized by a spectrum from indolent, polypoid tumors to sessile, more biologically aggressive lesions. Initial management relies heavily on cytoscopic procedures, but as disease becomes more advanced, imaging becomes central to decision making. This volume draws together contributions from various specialities, including pathology, surgery, and clinical and medical oncology. The aim is to inform the radiologist of the range of surgical procedures which has been developed, and the possibilities for management with radiotherapy. Cytotoxic chemotherapy can be used in neoadjuvant, adjuvant and palliative settings. The role of imaging in diagnosis of disease of the urothelium, the techniques for staging bladder cancer and detection of metastatic disease are each discussed in separate chapters. Imaging following treatment, including effects on normal tissues, is also covered, and the multidisciplinary nature of management of bladder neoplasms is emphasized. In line with the ethos of the *Contemporary Issues in Cancer Imaging* series, it is hoped that this volume will give radiologists a broader view of the technical aspects of treatment, and colleagues in other specialities will be able to further their understanding of the contribution imaging can make in our endeavors to cure the disease and control symptoms in patients with bladder cancer.

David MacVicar

1

The pathology of bladder cancer

Charles Jameson

Introduction

Carcinoma of the bladder is the seventh most common cancer worldwide [1]. It comprises 3.2% of all cancers, with an estimated 260 000 new cases each year in men and 76 000 in women. The highest incidence rates in males and females occur in Western Europe, North America and Australia. The UK annual incidence is over 10 000 new cases, with a male:female ratio of 5 : 2 [2–5].

Urothelial carcinoma is the most common type of bladder cancer. However, there is significant geographic variation, and in certain regions of the world, such as Egypt and parts of Africa, squamous cell carcinoma (SCC) of the bladder predominates.

Urothelial carcinomas of the renal pelvis, ureter and urethra are less common, accounting for approximately 10% of all urinary tract neoplasms.

It should be noted that the formerly used term "transitional cell carcinoma (TCC)" is now largely replaced by "urothelial carcinoma," although you will still hear urologists and pathologists use both interchangeably.

The WHO histological classification of tumors of the urinary tract (2004) is given in modified form in Table 1.1 [6].

The urothelium is the lining epithelium of the urinary collecting system and includes that of the renal pelvis, ureters, bladder and part of the urethra. Its thickness varies from three to seven cell layers, depending on the state of distension of the bladder. The turnover rate of those cells is low, of the order of three to six months. The cells desquamate but very few cells are seen in normal urine cytology specimens, i.e. normal urine is hypocellular. Very few mitotic figures are seen in normal urothelium. The presence of surface "umbrella cells" indicates normal maturation in the urothelium. These cells are large and elliptical and have abundant eosinophilic

Carcinoma of the Bladder, ed. David MacVicar. Published by Cambridge University Press. © Cambridge University Press 2008.

Table 1.1. WHO histological classification of tumors of the urinary tract [6] (modified)

Urothelial tumors

Infiltrating urothelial carcinoma
  with squamous differentiation
  with glandular differentiation
  micropapillary
  sarcomatoid

Non-invasive urothelial neoplasias
  urothelial carcinoma *in situ* (CIS)
  non-invasive papillary urothelial carcinoma, high grade
  non-invasive papillary urothelial carcinoma, low grade
  non-invasive papillary urothelial neoplasm of low malignant potential (PUNLMP)
  urothelial papilloma
  inverted urothelial papilloma

Squamous neoplasms
Squamous cell carcinoma
Verrucous carcinoma
Squamous cell papilloma

Glandular neoplasms
Adenocarcinoma
  enteric
  mucinous
  signet ring cell
Villous adenoma

Neuroendocrine tumors
Small cell carcinoma
Carcinoid
Paraganglioma

Melanocytic tumors
Malignant melanoma
Naevus

Mesenchymal tumors
Rhabdomyosarcoma
Leiomyosarcoma
Angiosarcoma
Other

Table 1.1. (cont.)

Urothelial tumors

Hemopoietic and lymphoid tumors
Lymphoma
Plasmacytoma

Miscellaneous tumors
Carcinoma of Skene, Cowper and Littre glands
Metastatic tumors and tumors extending from other organs

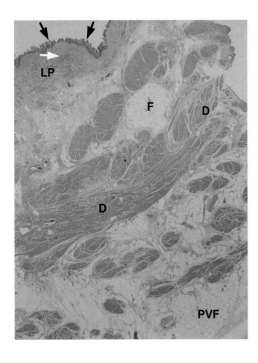

Figure 1.1 A section through normal bladder wall showing urothelium (arrows), lamina propria (LP), muscularis mucosae (white arrow), detrusor muscle (D) comprising inner longitudinal, circular, and outer longitudinal layers, and fat (F) distributed throughout wall. When tumor penetrates detrusor into perivesical fat (PVF) it becomes pT3 by TNM criteria (see also color plate section).

cytoplasm. The surface outline has a characteristic scalloped appearance. The umbrella cells have the unique property that they maintain the impermeability of the epithelium to urine, even when at full stretch. Figure 1.1 shows a section through a normal bladder wall and illustrates the urothelium, underlying lamina propria, muscularis mucosae, detrusor muscle and the perivesical fat. The thick muscle bundles of the detrusor may be difficult to distinguish and are distinct *only* in the region of the bladder neck. In addition, a thin, wispy, discontinuous layer of muscularis mucosae is present in about 5% of bladders and is located in the lamina propria. Fat can be present at all levels of the bladder wall.

Etiology

A number of risk factors are known for bladder cancer, of which smoking tobacco is the major one. Long-term use of analgesics containing phenacetin greatly increases the risk of developing urothelial cancer anywhere along the urinary collecting system. Occupational exposure to aniline dyes is also associated with bladder cancer. In particular, the aromatic amines benzidine and 2-naphthylamine and possibly 1-naphthylamine have been identified as bladder carcinogens. The drug cyclophosphamide has been reported to be associated with an increased risk of SCCs and sarcomas, particularly leiomyosarcomas. Chlornaphazine is also associated with bladder cancer development. In certain areas of the world schistosoma hematobium infections are associated with the development of SCCs of the bladder. Chronic infections and bladder calculi are also associated with these squamous tumors worldwide.

Genetics and multifocality of urothelial carcinomas

It is well known that urinary tract neoplasia is not necessarily limited to one single tumor. Frequent recurrence, multifocal tumors and the presence of "flat" lesions are characteristic of these tumors. Most multicentric bladder tumors are of monoclonal origin [6]. However, polyclonal cancers have also been reported [6], mainly in the early stages of tumors or in premalignant lesions. These observations have led to the hypothesis of "field defect," suggesting that environmental mutagens may cause fields of genetically altered cells that become the source of polyclonal, multifocal tumors [7].

Histopathological approach to bladder tumors

In histopathology practice, the types of specimens received from bladder cancers range from simple 3–4mm biopsies, to transurethral resection of (bladder) tumor (TURBT), to partial or radical cystectomy. In some cases cystoprostatectomy is performed and regional lymph node dissections may be performed for staging purposes.

There are a number of essential prognostic features to report in bladder tumor specimens, whether obtained as tumor biopsy samples (TURBT) or larger resection specimens (e.g. cystectomy), all of which have therapeutic import. These are as follows:

1. *Type of cancer*. Urothelial, squamous, and small cell carcinomas, adenocarcinoma, and other rarer types are all well described. Any variants of predominant tumor types and evidence of divergent differentiation should be noted.
2. *Grade*. This is a histological estimation of the degree of differentiation, in other words, how much a tumor resembles the tissue of origin. There are two main grading systems in use – most histopathologists and urologists still abide by the WHO 1973 grading system: grade 1 (well differentiated), grade 2 (moderately differentiated) and grade 3 (poorly differentiated). The future trend is to grade carcinomas as low grade or high grade, which is believed to be more relevant clinically. Grading is subjective by its nature and a more simple low/high grade approach reduces the interobserver variation considerably. The WHO 2004 grading system [6] incorporates the low/high grade approach.
3. *Stage*. The tumor, node, metastases (TNM) system (Table 1.2) is used in bladder cancer staging to describe pathological stage [8]. In TURBT specimens the pathologist is limited by the presence or absence of detrusor muscle tissue in the biopsy material. Often one can only say pT1b *at least*, e.g. if no muscle tissue is sampled in a carcinoma that invades the deep lamina propria. In biopsy samples where muscle is present, the stage could also be pT2a *at least*, as it is not possible to distinguish between the inner half of the muscularis (pT2a) and the outer half (pT2b).

   If a radical cystectomy is performed with lymph node sampling or dissection it is possible to give a much more complete pathological stage, e.g. pT4 N2 MX.

   Stage grouping is used by urologists, radiotherapists and oncologists once all the clinical, histopathological and radiological staging information is available [8]. Tumors of the renal pelvis, ureter and urethra have their own separate staging systems within the TNM system (Table 1.2).
4. *Diffuse or multifocal tumor*. It is important to describe the presence or absence of flat carcinoma *in situ* (CIS or pTis) in relation to the tumor itself or, more significantly, in random biopsy samples taken from the main tumor mass as the description has prognostic significance and impacts on management.
5. The presence or absence of detrusor muscle in the specimen.
6. *Lymphovascular (LVSI) space invasion*. This usually appears as small fragments of tumor in lymphatic spaces or blood vessels. It may also fill the vascular space completely as a so-called "tumor embolus." The significance of LVSI is in relation to possible tumor metastasis and is regarded by many oncologists as a poor prognostic factor.

The Royal College of Pathologists has produced a minimum dataset to incorporate all of the above features [9]. Tables 1.3, 1.4, and 1.5 illustrate the proformas for each specific urothelial tumor site.

Table 1.2. TNM pathological staging (6th edn, UICC)[8]

Renal pelvis and ureter

pT – Primary tumor

pTX   Primary tumor cannot be assessed

pT0   No evidence of primary tumor

pTa   Non-invasive papillary carcinoma

pTis   Carcinoma *in situ*

pT1   Tumor invades subepithelial connective tissue

pT2   Tumor invades muscularis

pT3   (Renal pelvis) Tumor invades beyond muscularis into peripelvic fat or renal parenchyma
       (Ureter) Tumor invades beyond muscularis into periureteric fat

pT4   Tumor invades adjacent organs or through the kidney into perinephric fat

pN – Regional lymph nodes

pNX   Regional lymph nodes cannot be assessed

pN0   No regional lymph node metastasis

pN1   Metastasis in a single lymph node 2 cm or less in greatest dimension

pN2   Metastasis in a single lymph node more than 2 cm but not more than 5 cm in greatest
       dimension, or multiple lymph nodes, none more than 5 cm in greatest dimension

pN3   Metastasis in a lymph node more than 5 cm in greatest dimension

pM – Distant metastases

pMX   Distant metastases cannot be assessed

pM0   No distant metastasis

pM1   Distant metastases

Stage grouping

Stage 0a	Ta	N0	M0
Stage 0is	Tis	N0	M0
Stage I	T1	N0	M0
Stage II	T2	N0	M0
Stage III	T3	N0	M0
Stage IV	T4	N0	M0
	Any T	N1, N2, N3	M0
	Any T	Any N	M1

Urinary bladder

pT – Primary tumor

pTX   Primary tumor cannot be assessed

pT0   No evidence of primary tumor

pTa   Non-invasive papillary carcinoma

pTis   Carcinoma *in situ*

Table 1.2. (cont.)

pT1   Tumor invades subepithelial connective tissue
pT2   Tumor invades muscle:
pT2a   Tumor invades superficial muscle (inner half)
pT2b   Tumor invades deep muscle (outer half)
pT3   Tumor invades perivesical tissue:
pT3a   microscopically
pT3b   macroscopically (extravesical mass)
pT4   Tumor invades any of the following: prostate, uterus, vagina, pelvic wall, abdominal wall:
pT4a   Tumor invades prostate, uterus or vagina
pT4b   Tumor invades pelvic wall or abdominal wall

pN – Regional lymph nodes
pNX   Regional lymph nodes cannot be assessed
pN0   No regional lymph node metastasis
pN1   Metastasis in a single lymph node 2 cm or less in greatest dimension
pN2   Metastasis in a single lymph node more than 2 cm but not more than 5 cm in greatest
            dimension, or multiple lymph nodes, none more than 5 cm in greatest dimension
pN3   Metastasis in a lymph node more than 5 cm in greatest dimension

pM – Distant metastases
pMX   Distant metastases cannot be assessed
pM0   No distant metastasis
pM1   Distant metastases

Stage grouping

Stage 0a	Ta	N0	M0
Stage 0is	Tis	N0	M0
Stage I	T1	N0	M0
Stage II	T2a,b	N0	M0
Stage III	T3a,b	N0	M0
	T4a	N0	M0
Stage IV	T4b	N0	M0
	Any T	N1, N2, N3	M0
	Any T	Any N	M1

Urethra
pT –   Primary tumor
pTX   Primary tumor cannot be assessed
pT0   No evidence of primary tumor
Male and female
pTa   Non-invasive papillary, polypoid or verrucous carcinoma

Table 1.2. (cont.)

pTis	Carcinoma *in situ*
pT1	Tumor invades subepithelial connective tissue
pT2	Tumor invades any of the following: corpus spongiosum, prostate, periurethral muscle
pT3	Tumor invades any of the following: corpus cavernosum, beyond prostatic capsule, anterior vagina, bladder neck
pT4	Tumor invades other adjacent organs

Transitional cell carcinoma of the prostate (prostatic urethra)

pTis pu	Carcinoma *in situ*, involvement of prostatic urethra
pTis pd	Carcinoma *in situ*, involvement of prostatic ducts
pT1	Tumor invades subepithelial connective tissue
pT2	Tumor invades any of the following: prostatic stroma, corpus spongiosum, periurethral muscle
pT3	Tumor invades any of the following: corpus cavernosum, beyond prostatic capsule, bladder neck (extraprostatic extension)
pT4	Tumor invades other adjacent organs (invasion of bladder)

pN –	**Regional lymph nodes**
pNx	Regional lymph nodes cannot be assessed
pN0	No regional lymph node metastasis
pN1	Metastasis in a single lymph node 2 cm or less in greatest dimension
pN2	Metastasis in a single lymph node more than 2 cm or multiple lymph nodes

pM –	**Distant metastases**
pMX	Distant metastases cannot be assessed
pM0	No distant metastasis
pM1	Distant metastases

Stage grouping

Stage 0a	Ta	N0	M0
Stage 0is	Tis	N0	M0
	Tis pu	N0	M0
	Tis pd	N0	M0
Stage I	T1	N0	M0
Stage II	T2	N0	M0
Stage III	T1, T2	N1	M0
	T3	N0, N1	M0
Stage IV	T4	N0, N1	M0
	Any T	N2	M0
	Any T	Any N	M1

Table 1.3. Reporting proforma: urinary bladder

Surname............................ Forenames.........................
Date of birth............ Sex....
Hospital............................ Hospital no. ....
NHS no..................
Date of receipt................... Date of reporting...................
Report no...............
Pathologist......................... Surgeon...........................

Nature of specimen/procedure and core macroscopic items

Biopsy ☐ TURBT ☐ Diverticulectomy ☐ Partial cystectomy ☐ **Radical cystectomy** ☐
Site(s) of biopsy or TURBT.......................... Tumor location.....................

Weight of TURBT.............................(g) Maximum tumor size ... (mm)
Number of tumors.................
Right obturator nodes Yes ☐ No ☐ Left obturator nodes Yes ☐ No ☐
Right pelvic nodes Yes ☐ No ☐ Left pelvic nodes Yes ☐ No ☐

Invasion into perivesical tissue (pT3b) Yes ☐ No ☐ Cannot assess ☐

Margins N/A ☐ Negative ☐ Positive ☐
Distance to the nearest margin ....(mm) Site(s)......

Core microscopic items

Tumor subtype (s) (one or more)	Urothelial carcinoma ☐	For urothelial carcinomas:	WHO 1973	WHO 2004
	Squamous carcinoma ☐		Grade 1 ☐	Low grade ☐
	Adenocarcinoma ☐		Grade 2 ☐	
	Small cell carcinoma ☐			High grade ☐
	Sarcomatoid carcinoma ☐		Grade 3 ☐	
	Sarcoma ☐			
	Other: ☐	Associated CIS	Yes ☐ No ☐	
	Please specify:....................	Vascular invasion	Yes ☐ No ☐	

Carcinoma *in situ* only (pTis) Yes ☐ No ☐ Cannot assess (pTx) ☐
Non-invasive papillary tumor (pTa) Yes ☐ No ☐ Cannot assess (pTx) ☐
Invasion into lamina propria (pT1) Yes ☐ No ☐ Cannot assess (pTx) ☐
Invasion into inner half of muscle (pT2a) Yes ☐ No ☐ Cannot assess (pTx) ☐
Invasion into outer half of muscle (pT2b) Yes ☐ No ☐ Cannot assess (pTx) ☐
Microscopic invasion into perivesical tissue (pT3a) Yes ☐ No ☐ Cannot assess (pTx) ☐
Invasion into perivesical tissue confirmed (pT3b) Yes ☐ No ☐ Cannot assess (pTx) ☐
Invasion into prostate, uterus, or vagina (pT4a) Yes ☐ No ☐ Cannot assess (pTx) ☐
Invasion into pelvic or abdominal wall (pT4b) Yes ☐ No ☐ Cannot assess (pTx) ☐

Margins N/A ☐ Negative ☐ Positive ☐
Distance to the nearest margin ....(mm) Site(s).................

Right nodes	Total	No pos	ECS		Left nodes	Total	No pos	ECS	
Obturator				N/A ☐	Obturator				N/A ☐
Pelvic				N/A ☐	Pelvic				N/A ☐
Other:				N/A ☐	Other:				N/A ☐
Please specify...........................					Please specify...........................				

pTNM stage: pT .... pN......... pM....... SNOMED codes
T................... M.....................
T................... M.....................

Signature of pathologist... Date.......................

Table 1.4. Reporting proforma: renal pelvis and ureter

Surname...........................   Forenames.........................
Date of birth............   Sex....
Hospital...........................   Hospital no........................
NHS no..................
Date of receipt...................   Date of reporting................
Report no...............
Pathologist........................   Surgeon...........................

Nature of specimen/procedure and core macroscopic items

Biopsy ☐   Right ☐   Left ☐   Right ☐   Left nephroureterectomy ☐
                    ureter   ureter   nephroureterectomy
Site(s) of biopsy ....   Tumor location ....
                                Number of tumors......
                                Maximum tumor size ....(mm)
Nodes   Yes ☐   No ☐
Please specify origin...............

Margins   N/A ☐   Negative ☐   Positive ☐
                Distance to the nearest margin ....(mm)   Site(s).................

Core microscopic items

Tumor subtype (s) (one or more)	Urothelial carcinoma ☐	**For urothelial carcinomas:**	**WHO 1973**		WHO 2004	
	Squamous carcinoma ☐		Grade 1 ☐		Low grade ☐	
	Adenocarcinoma ☐		Grade 2 ☐			
	Small cell carcinoma ☐				High grade ☐	
	Sarcomatoid carcinoma ☐		Grade 3 ☐			
	Sarcoma ☐					
	Other: ☐	Associated CIS	Yes ☐ No ☐			
	Please specify:....................	Vascular invasion	Yes ☐ No ☐			

Carcinoma *in situ* only (pTis)   Yes ☐ No ☐ Cannot assess (pTx) ☐
Non-invasive papillary tumor (pTa)   Yes ☐ No ☐ Cannot assess (pTx) ☐
Invasion into subepithelial connective tissue (pT1)   Yes ☐ No ☐ Cannot assess (pTx) ☐
Invasion into muscularis (pT2)   Yes ☐ No ☐ Cannot assess (pTx) ☐
(Renal pelvis) Invasion into renal peripelvic fat or renal parenchyma (pT3)   Yes ☐ No ☐ Cannot assess (pTx) ☐
(Ureter) Invasion into periureteric fat (pT3)   Yes ☐ No ☐ Cannot assess (pTx) ☐
Invasion into adjacent organs or through kidney to perinephric fat (pT4)   Yes ☐ No ☐ Cannot assess (pTx) ☐

Margins   N/A ☐   Negative ☐   Positive ☐
                Distance to the nearest margin ....(mm)   Site(s).................

Nodes   N/A ☐   Total   No positive   ECS   Yes ☐ No ☐
Origin:

pTNM stage: pT .... pN......... pM.......   SNOMED codes
                                T................... M...................
                                T................... M...................

Signature of pathologist..
Date.....................

Table 1.5. Reporting proforma: urethra

Surname...........................   Forenames.........................
Date of birth............   Sex....
Hospital...........................   Hospital no.........................
NHS no..................
Date of receipt...................   Date of reporting.................
Report no...............
Pathologist........................   Surgeon...........................

Nature of specimen/procedure and core macroscopic items

Biopsy ☐   TURT ☐   Diverticulectomy ☐   Urethrectomy ☐
Site(s) of biopsy or TURT......................... Tumor location......................
Weight of TURT.................(g)   Number of tumors.................
    Maximum tumor size ....(mm)

Nodes   Yes ☐   No ☐
Please specify origin...............

Margins   **N/A** ☐   **Negative** ☐   **Positive** ☐
    Distance to the nearest margin ....(mm)   Site(s).................

Core microscopic items

Tumor subtype(s) (one or more)				**For urothelial carcinomas:**	**WHO 1973**		__WHO 2004	
Urothelial carcinoma	☐				Grade 1	☐	Low grade	☐
Squamous carcinoma	☐				Grade 2	☐		
Adenocarcinoma	☐						High grade	☐
Small cell carcinoma	☐							
Sarcomatoid carcinoma	☐				Grade 3	☐		
Sarcoma	☐							
Other:	☐			Associated CIS	Yes ☐	No ☐		
Please specify:....................				Vascular invasion	Yes ☐	No ☐		

	Yes	No	Cannot assess (pTx)	
Carcinoma *in situ* only (pTis, add pu or pd if prostatic urethral or ducts)	☐	☐	☐	☐
Non-invasive papillary tumor (pTa)	☐	☐	☐	☐
Invasion into subepithelial connective tissue (pT1)	☐	☐	☐	☐
Invasion into corpus spongiosum, prostate, periurethral muscle (pT2)	☐	☐	☐	☐
Invasion into corpus cavernosum, beyond prostatic capsule, anterior vagina, bladder neck (pT3)	☐	☐	☐	☐
Invasion into other adjacent organs (pT4)	☐	☐	☐	☐

Margins   **N/A** ☐   **Negative** ☐   **Positive** ☐
    Distance to the nearest margin ....(mm)   Site(s).................

Nodes   N/A ☐   Total   No positive   ECS   Yes ☐   No ☐
Origin:

pTNM stage: pT .... pN......... pM.......   SNOMED codes
       T................... M.......................
       T................... M.......................

Signature of pathologist..   Date......................

Many, but not all, laboratories produce a formatted report which incorporates all of the significant features for a particular tumor site in a "tick box" scheme. This has the advantage over text reporting in that certain "minimum" criteria in a cancer report are not omitted. Most laboratories also have a free text section to include other specific details which are not covered in the minimum dataset, e.g. resection margin measurements.

Benign and low malignant potential urothelial lesions

Urothelial papilloma

This lesion consists of frond-like projections with a central fibrovascular core and is lined by urothelium resembling normal urothelium. They are usually single tumors and rarely recur. They are not distinguishable cystoscopically from papillary urothelial neoplasms of low malignant potential (PUNLMP) or low grade papillary urothelial carcinoma.

Inverted papilloma

This is a benign tumor which exhibits an inverted growth pattern. It has minimal cytological atypia. Recurrence is rare and progression to urothelial carcinomas is even rarer.

Papillary urothelial neoplasms of low malignant potential (PUNLMP)

This lesion is a papillary tumor of urothelium which morphologically resembles its benign papilloma counterpart, but which shows increased cellular proliferation which exceeds the thickness of normal urothelium [6]. Its existence is somewhat controversial as distinguishing this lesion from a benign papilloma or a low grade papillary urothelial carcinoma generates considerable interobserver variation among pathologists. The lesion may recur but less often than low grade non-invasive papillary urothelial carcinomas.

Urothelial carcinoma

The vast majority of cancers arising in the urinary tract are of urothelial origin. These can be divided into four broad categories:

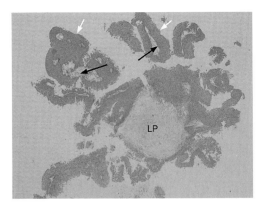

Figure 1.2 The typical biopsy appearances of a low grade papillary urothelial carcinoma (stage pTa), showing frond-like projections. These have a central fibrovascular core (black arrows) and thickened malignant urothelium surrounding it (white arrows). Lamina propria (LP) is present in the specimen. The cystoscopist will readily recognize the papillary growth pattern (see also color plate section).

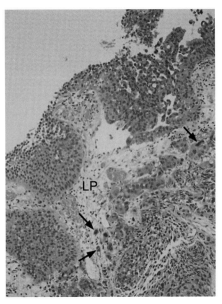

Figure 1.3 This shows invasion of the lamina propria (LP) by a high grade urothelial carcinoma (stage pT1). Some clusters of very atypical cells with large hyperchromatic nuclei are present (arrows). The growth pattern is irregular (see also color plate section).

Papillary, superficial (non-invasive) tumors *or* minimally invasive tumors

These are usually of low grade and are visible in most cases cystoscopically as frond-like projections on the bladder surface. Typical biopsy appearances are shown in Figures 1.2 and 1.3. They are *not* normally visible when radiological imaging techniques are used.

Invasive carcinomas

These may be non-papillary or with papillary areas. Those that invade the detrusor muscle of the bladder and beyond are usually of high grade. They can show a variety of macroscopic appearances and can be exophytic, polypoid, endophytic and ulcerated. These tumors *are* normally visible when radiological imaging techniques are used. Figure 1.4 demonstrates the gross morphology of a urothelial carcinoma of endophytic growth pattern and Figure 1.5 shows the histological appearance of a urothelial carcinoma corresponding to such a tumor.

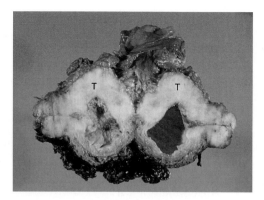

Figure 1.4 This shows a bladder containing a urothelial carcinoma (T) that is diffusely infiltrating and thickening the bladder wall (endophytic growth pattern). This should be readily visible with cross-sectional imaging (see also color plate section).

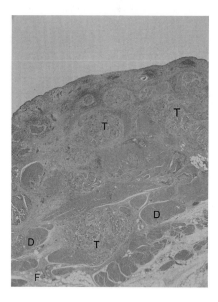

Figure 1.5 The histological appearances of the tumor in Figure 1.4. Carcinoma (T) extends right through the wall of the bladder, dissecting and destroying detrusor muscle (D). It also extended into perivesical fat (F) (stage pT3). This endophytic solid growth pattern can leave the urothelium intact with no formation of papillae (see also color plate section).

Flat carcinoma *in situ* (CIS)

This is a high grade urothelial lesion. This is only seen cystoscopically as a flat red patch or patches. Figure 1.6 shows the typical histological appearance.

About 70% of bladder tumors are non-invasive (pTa) or invade the lamina propria only (pT1a or pT1b). Urologists often refer to both types as "superficial tumors." Only about 5% of pTa and 20% of pT1 carcinomas go on to invade the deep muscle of the bladder, with consequent metastatic potential [10]. Muscle-invasive cancers are usually invasive from the outset, only 10–20% being preceded by lower stage carcinomas [11].

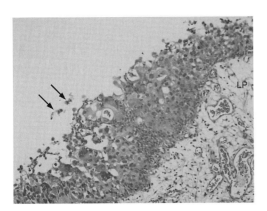

Figure 1.6 Flat carcinoma *in situ* (CIS). Full thickness atypia with dyscohesive cells (arrows) falling away from the surface are typical. There is no invasion into lamina propria (LP) (see also color plate section).

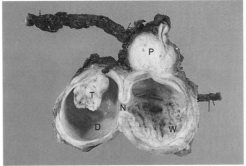

Figure 1.7 A urothelial carcinoma (T) arising in a bladder diverticulum (D). It is easy for a cystoscopist to miss such a tumor if the neck (N) is narrow. The bladder wall (W) is trabeculated probably as a result of prostatic (P) enlargement (see also color plate section).

Carcinoma *in situ* is a high grade flat lesion, most of which will progress to invasive carcinomas if not treated [12]. Treatment is with BCG therapy initially, which may induce a granulomatous cystitis afterwards.

Variants of urothelial carcinoma

Variant types of urothelial carcinoma are set out in Table 1.1. These are normally tumors which show prominent areas of differentiation toward squamous, glandular or other types of carcinoma, but in which the primary diagnosis is still "urothelial carcinoma." It has been suggested that these variants are more resistant to radiotherapy (especially the squamous variant) and chemotherapy, but the evidence is not conclusive. They should be noted in the free text section of histopathology reports.

Urothelial carcinomas are also known to occur in bladder diverticula (Fig. 1.7), along with squamous carcinomas.

Squamous cell carcinoma

This is a carcinoma of urothelial lining origin showing pure squamous morphology throughout. It differs from urothelial carcinoma showing squamous differentiation, which should primarily be regarded as a urothelial malignancy, by virtue of histological appearance and, often, growth pattern.

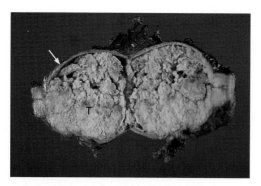

Figure 1.8 The gross appearances of a bulky squamous cell carcinoma of bladder with tumor filling the bladder lumen. The bladder wall remains thin (arrow), while the tumor (T) shows an exophytic growth pattern (compare with Fig. 1.4) (see also color plate section).

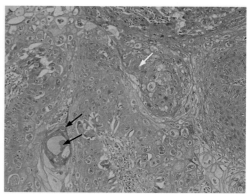

Figure 1.9 The microscopic appearances of a squamous cell carcinoma – note the keratin production (black arrows) by this tumor forming "keratin pearls" in places (white arrow). No normal bladder wall tissue is present on this section (see also color plate section).

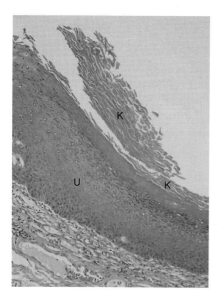

Figure 1.10 Keratinizing squamous metaplasia of the bladder. The urothelium (U) has thickened and the individual cells now have the appearance of squamous cells. Layers of keratin (K) have been produced, which have a white appearance on cystoscopy (see also color plate section).

The geographical variation in the incidence of bladder SCC primarily relates to schistosomal infections. Thus, Egypt, West Africa and South-east Africa have higher incidences of SCC than urothelial carcinomas. In South Africa there is an interracial difference in the histology [13]. In black patients the percentage of bladder tumors is 36% SCC and 41% urothelial tumors; in white patients it is 2% SCC and 94% urothelial.

The associations of SCC of the bladder are *Schistosoma haematobium* infections, pre-existing keratinizing squamous metaplasia and chronic irritation due to stones or chronic cystitis.

Most squamous carcinomas are polypoid, bulky, ulcerated and fill the bladder lumen (Fig. 1.8). Normally a large amount of keratin and necrotic material is present on the surface. The larger tumors are normally seen when radiological imaging techniques are used.

The histology varies from the well-differentiated keratinizing type (Fig. 1.9) to poorly differentiated forms with no keratin formation. The non-tumor areas of the bladder may show evidence of pre-existing keratinizing squamous metaplasia (Fig. 1.10) and/or SCC *in situ*.

Adenocarcinoma

This is a malignant tumor of urothelial origin showing gland formation throughout (Fig. 1.11). It differs from urothelial carcinomas showing adenoid (glandular) differentiation, again which should be regarded as primarily urothelial carcinomas.

It is an uncommon tumor of the bladder, accounting for approximately 2% of all bladder cancers. It includes primary adenocarcinoma of the bladder *and* urachal carcinoma. Metastatic spread of adenocarcinoma from other sites, most often rectum and prostate, is *much more common* than primary bladder adenocarcinomas. Figure 1.12 shows direct spread of metastatic adenocarcinoma of prostate

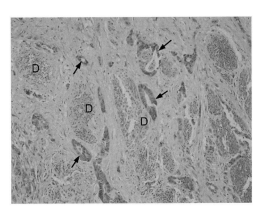

Figure 1.11 Adenocarcinoma infiltrating between detrusor muscle fibers (D) of the bladder wall. Gland formation characterizes the tumor (arrows) (see also color plate section).

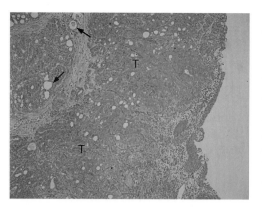

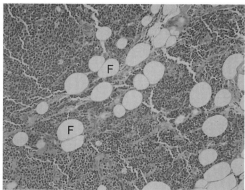

Figure 1.12 Metastatic adenocarcinoma of prostate (T) with prominent gland formation (arrows). Normal bladder wall structures are not seen (see also color plate section).

Figure 1.13 Small cell carcinoma of bladder infiltrates the perivesical fat (F). The malignant cells are small and lymphocyte-like, forming a diffuse sheet of tumor (see also color plate section).

invading the bladder wall. Transcoelomic spread of colonic and gastric cancer to the bladder is also seen but is rare.

The majority of adenocarcinoma of the bladder are associated with long-standing intestinal (colonic type) metaplasia of the urothelium. Thus, patients with non-functioning bladders owing to bladder extrophy, obstruction, cystocoele, and chronic irritation are most at risk of developing this tumor [6].

Urachal carcinomas arise in urachal remnants of the bladder and are most commonly located in the dome and the anterior wall. They occur less frequently in the posterior wall and they extend to the umbilicus. Adenocarcinomas are the most common, with squamous and other types also occurring.

Small cell (neuroendocrine) carcinoma

These are carcinomas derived from the urothelium and which morphologically resemble their lung counterparts. They occur almost exclusively in the bladder and prostate rather than elsewhere in the urinary tract, with the bladder being the commonest site. They appear as large, solid, polypoid masses with or without ulceration and often extensively infiltrate the wall of the bladder by the time of presentation (Fig. 1.13). They are very aggressive cancers with vascular and detrusor muscle invasion. The importance of diagnosing this type of carcinoma lies in its response to chemotherapy.

The neuroendocrine nature of these tumors is identified in the immunohisto-chemical stains performed to confirm the diagnosis, e.g. CD56, chromogranin and synaptophysin.

Metastatic small cell carcinomas from other sites need to be considered in the clinical differential diagnosis of these malignancies.

Rare cancers and benign tumors of the bladder

There are a wide variety of uncommon benign tumors which may occur along the urinary tract, such as a leiomyoma. A list of these is given in the WHO histological classification (Table 1.1). The most common site for these is the bladder, and less often the urethra.

Rare bladder malignancies include malignant melanoma, lymphoma, and soft tissue sarcomas. These are diagnosed by biopsy and immunohistochemical markers.

Metastatic cancers to the bladder

These are tumors of non-urothelial origin extending to the bladder, most often in the region of the bladder neck and trigone. The commonest primary sites are prostate, colorectum and uterine cervix. Less common primaries include stomach, skin, breast and lung.

Histologically these cancers often underrun the urothelium. There is no asso-ciated flat CIS with these tumors. Immunohistochemical staining patterns gener-ally differ from those of primary urothelial carcinomas, raising the question of metastasis, which has obvious clinical and pathological significance.

Tumors of the renal pelvis and ureter

Tumors of the renal pelvis account for 8% of all urinary tract neoplasms and 90% of these are urothelial carcinomas [14]. Renal pelvic tumors are twice as common as those of the ureter. Multifocality is frequent. The majority of these carcinomas arise following diagnosis of a bladder tumor. They often present with hematuria and flank pain. Once a diagnosis of urothelial bladder cancer has been made, the index of suspicion for further neoplasms in the urinary tract should remain high.

The cancers tend to be papillary and very often low grade, but may also be polypoid, ulcerative, infiltrative and high grade. Some tumors distend the whole of

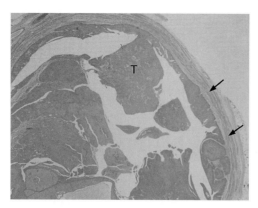

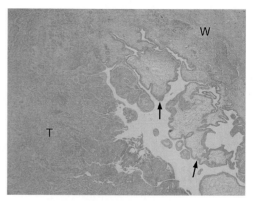

Figure 1.14 A dilated ureter containing papillary low grade urothelial tumor of exophytic growth pattern (T). Muscle layers in the ureteric wall are preserved (arrows) (see also color plate section).

Figure 1.15 Urothelial carcinoma of renal pelvis. Normal wall is present (W), with tumor showing areas of papillary growth (arrows) and a more solid mass (T) infiltrating underlying tissues (see also color plate section).

the renal pelvis in a very exophytic growth pattern. Hydronephrosis is sometimes the presenting clinical sign radiologically.

The ureter may appear dilated due to the lumen filling with exophytic tumor (Fig. 1.14), producing a hydronephrosis. Figure 1.15 shows a urothelial carcinoma of the renal pelvis.

The WHO grading of carcinomas of the renal pelvis and ureter is the same as for bladder urothelial carcinomas but there are separate TNM staging systems for these tumors (Table 1.2).

Squamous carcinomas, adenocarcinomas and rarer non-epithelial tumors may also arise at these sites but are very much less frequent than in the bladder.

Tumors of the urethra

These account for approximately 2% of all urinary tract neoplasms.

Urethral carcinomas are commonly associated with chronic human papillomavirus (HPV) infection. The lesions include squamous cell papillomas, which may show evidence of HPV histologically; squamous carcinomas; urothelial carcinomas; and less commonly adenocarcinomas. Carcinoma *in situ* may also be seen in the urethra.

The typical histological appearance of a urethral carcinoma (urothelial) is shown in Figure 1.16.

The tumors macroscopically may be papillary, polypoid, nodular, ulcerated or infiltrative, just like their bladder counterparts.

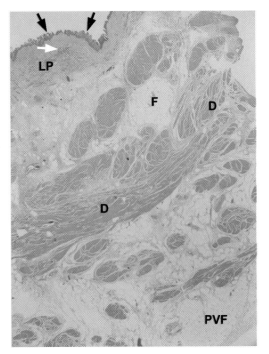

Figure 1.1 A section through normal bladder wall showing urothelium (arrows), lamina propria (LP), muscularis mucosae (white arrow), detrusor muscle (D) comprising inner longitudinal, circular, and outer longitudinal layers, and fat (F) distributed throughout wall. When tumor penetrates detrusor into perivesical fat (PVF) it becomes pT3 by TNM criteria.

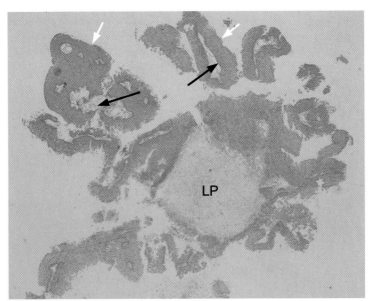

Figure 1.2 The typical biopsy appearances of a low grade papillary urothelial carcinoma (stage pTa), showing frond-like projections. These have a central fibrovascular core (black arrows) and thickened malignant urothelium surrounding it (white arrows). Lamina propria (LP) is present in the specimen. The cystoscopist will readily recognize the papillary growth pattern.

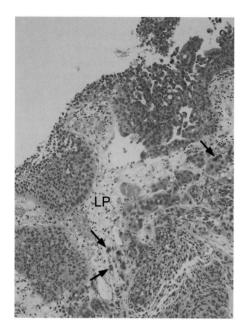

Figure 1.3 This shows invasion of the lamina propria (LP) by a high grade urothelial carcinoma (stage pT1). Some clusters of very atypical cells with large hyperchromatic nuclei are present (arrows). The growth pattern is irregular.

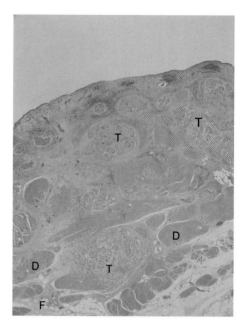

Figure 1.5 The histological appearances of the tumor in Figure 1.4. Carcinoma (T) extends right through the wall of the bladder, dissecting and destroying detrusor muscle (D). It also extended into perivesical fat (F) (stage pT3). This endophytic solid growth pattern can leave the urothelium intact with no formation of papillae.

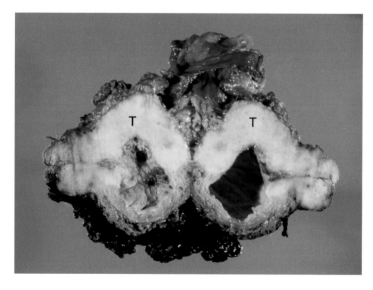

Figure 1.4 This shows a bladder containing a urothelial carcinoma (T) that is diffusely infiltrating and thickening the bladder wall (endophytic growth pattern). This should be readily visible with cross-sectional imaging.

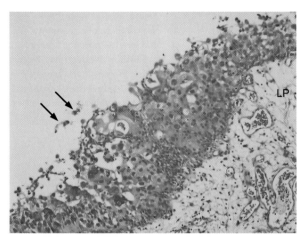

Figure 1.6 Flat carcinoma *in situ* (CIS). Full thickness atypia with dyscohesive cells (arrows) falling away from the surface are typical. There is no invasion into lamina propria (LP).

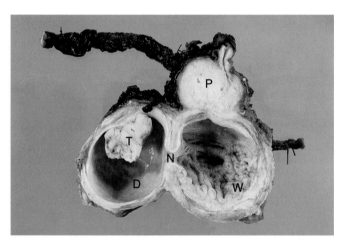

Figure 1.7 A urothelial carcinoma (T) arising in a bladder diverticulum (D). It is easy for a cystoscopist to miss such a tumor if the neck (N) is narrow. The bladder wall (W) is trabeculated probably as a result of prostatic (P) enlargement.

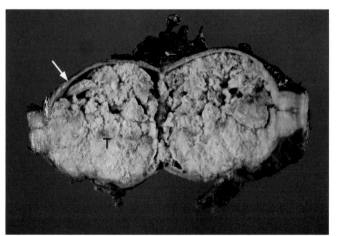

Figure 1.8 The gross appearances of a bulky squamous cell carcinoma of bladder with tumor filling the bladder lumen. The bladder wall remains thin (arrow), while the tumor (T) shows an exophytic growth pattern (compare with Figure 1.4).

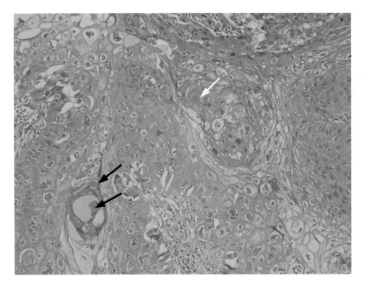

Figure 1.9 The microscopic appearances of a squamous cell carcinoma – note the keratin production (black arrows) by this tumor forming "keratin pearls" in places (white arrow). No normal bladder wall tissue is present on this section.

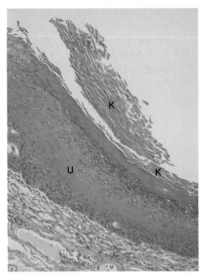

Figure 1.10 Keratinizing squamous metaplasia of the bladder. The urothelium (U) has thickened and the individual cells now have the appearance of squamous cells. Layers of keratin (K) have been produced, which have a white appearance on cystoscopy.

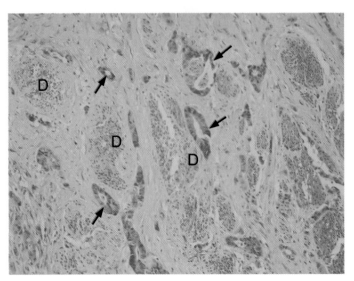

Figure 1.11 Adenocarcinoma infiltrating between detrusor muscle fibers (D) of the bladder wall. Gland formation characterizes the tumor (arrows).

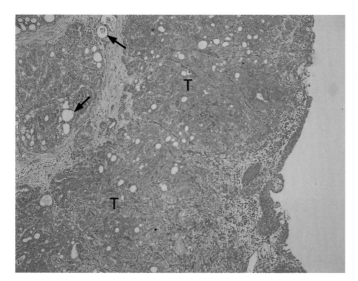

Figure 1.12 Metastatic adenocarcinoma of prostate (T) with prominent gland formation (arrows). Normal bladder wall structures are not seen.

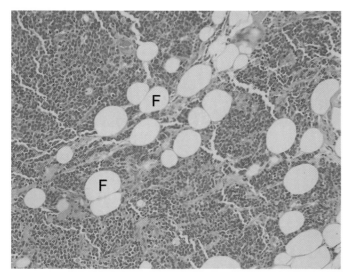

Figure 1.13 Small cell carcinoma of bladder infiltrates the perivesical fat (F). The malignant cells are small and lymphocyte-like, forming a diffuse sheet of tumor.

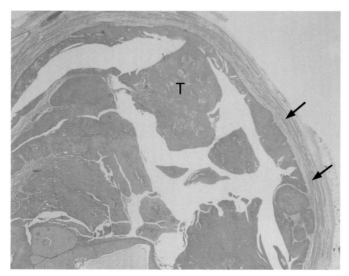

Figure 1.14 A dilated ureter containing papillary low grade urothelial tumor of exophytic growth pattern (T). Muscle layers in the ureteric wall are preserved (arrows).

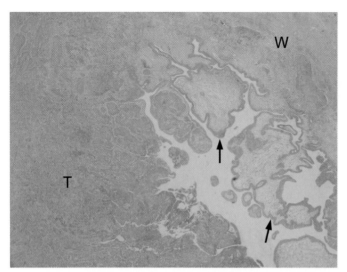

Figure 1.15 Urothelial carcinoma of renal pelvis. Normal wall is present (W), with tumor showing areas of papillary growth (arrows) and a more solid mass (T) infiltrating underlying tissues.

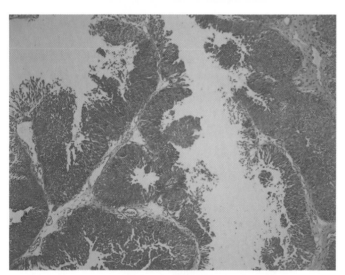

Figure 1.16 A papillary urothelial carcinoma of urethra similar to the appearance of bladder carcinoma (compare with Fig. 1.2).

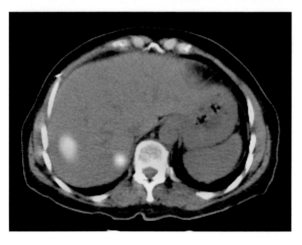

Figure 5.4 (c) Fused axial FDG PET-CT images reveal avid FDG uptake within metabolically active metastases from urothelial neoplasm within the right lobe of the liver.

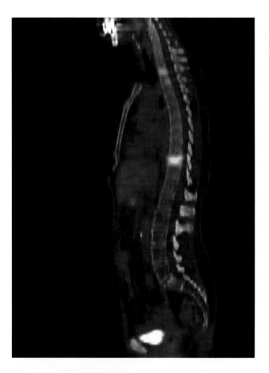

Figure 5.6 (b) Fused sagittal FDG PET-CT confirms the presence of metabolically active metastases within the vertebrae.

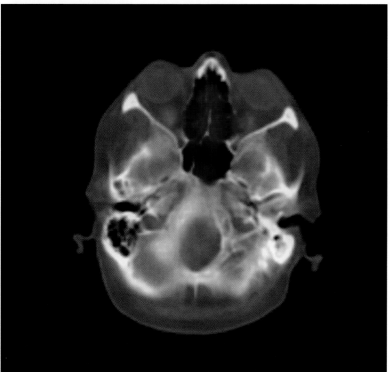

Figure 5.8 In a patient with known metastatic urothelial cancer to the liver and bones, fused axial FDG PET-CT demonstrates avid FDG uptake within a radiographically occult metastasis within the right skull base to be the cause for the patient's symptoms.

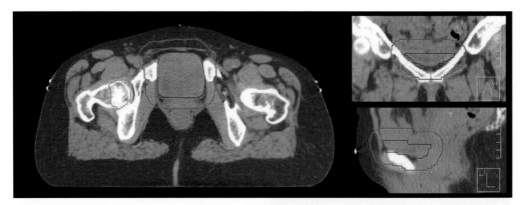

Figure 7.1 Axial, coronal and sagittal views of CT planning scan with clinical target volume (CTV) (blue) and planning target volume (PTV) (magenta) contoured.

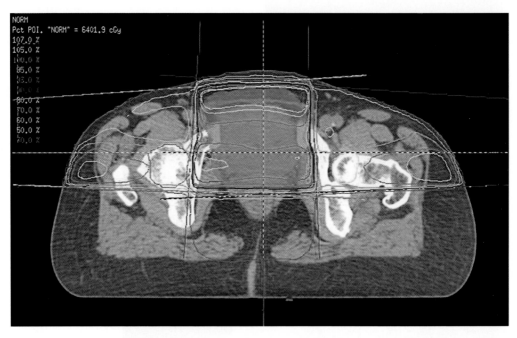

Figure 7.2 The margins of the three fields are outlined by red lines (AP field) at green and blue lines (lateral field). The planning target volume (PTV), shaded magenta, is placed over the area to be treated. Within this area the dose should be 95–105% of the dose at the isocenter of the volume. Each colored line represents an area of dose expressed as a percentage of the dose at the isocenter of PTV. These dose estimations are calculated from data acquired from phantom studies.

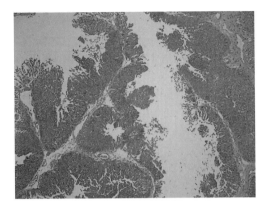

Figure 1.16 A papillary urothelial carcinoma of urethra similar to the appearance of bladder carcinoma (compare with Fig. 1.2) (see also color plate section).

The histological grading of these tumors is similar to that of the bladder tumors but the TNM staging system is once again different for urethral tumors (Table 1.2).

A note on urinary cytology

Cytological analysis of urine samples done with a view to cancer diagnosis needs some degree of caution with respect to interpretation. Because the lower grade urothelial carcinoma cells may appear very bland (minimal pleomorphism, no mitotic figures) in cytology preparations, it is not always possible to exclude these tumors on routine cytology. Patients with high grade carcinomas and flat CIS, however, generally give a much better yield of "malignant cytology" reports. In short, the sensitivity of urine cytology is low, but the positive predictive values for high grade carcinomas and flat CIS from urine samples sent for cytology are high.

Conclusion

Bladder cancer is a very good example of a "diverse" malignancy – geographical variations in tumor type, known risk factors in its causation, multifocality, high grade flat lesions, frequent recurrence, variable cystoscopic, radiological and histopathological appearances all demonstrate the heterogeneity of these cancers.

In the Western world the vast majority of bladder cancers are urothelial (transitional cell) carcinomas. In addition, flat CIS of the bladder requires aggressive management from its initial diagnosis in order to prevent invasive malignancy. The grading and staging of these tumors is crucial in the adequate management of patients with these malignancies. This necessitates both essential pathological and radiological input from the tumor's initial diagnosis.

The future of bladder cancer diagnosis requires differentiating those low grade non-aggressive tumors, which may not even recur once treated, from the aggressive, high grade tumors and high grade flat CIS. In the future, molecular pathology might be able to do this for us. Until then, light microscopy is to be regarded as the gold standard.

REFERENCES

1. Ferlay J, Bray F, Pisani P, Parkin D M. *GLOBOCAN 2000: Cancer Incidence, Mortality and Prevalence Worldwide.* Lyon: IARC Press, 2001.
2. Office for National Statistics. *Cancer Statistics Registrations: Registrations of Cancer Diagnosed in 2003, England.* Series MB1 No. 34. Vol. 2006, London: National Statistics.
3. Welsh Cancer Intelligence and Surveillance Unit (www.wales.nhs.uk).
4. Cancer incidence and mortality data; ISD Online. Cancer Research UK (http://info.cancerre searchuk.org/cancerstats).
5. Northern Ireland Cancer Registry. Cancer statistics (www.qub.ac.uk/research-centres).
6. Eble J N, Sauter G, Epstein J I, Sesterhenn I A (eds.). *World Health Organization Classification of Tumours. Pathology and Genetics of Tumours of the Urinary System and Male Genital Tract Organs.* Lyon: IARC Press, 2004.
7. Koss L G. Mapping of the urinary bladder: its impact on the concept of bladder cancer. *Hum Pathol* 1979; **10**: 533–48.
8. Sobin L H, Wittekind C. *TNM Classification of Malignant Tumours* (6th edn). New York: Wiley-Liss, 2002.
9. Dataset for tumours of the urinary collecting system (Renal pelvis, ureter, bladder and urethra). Coordinators: Dr. Patricia Harnden, Professor Richard Ball, Dr. Alex Freeman, University College London, January 2007.
10. Minimum Dataset for Bladder Tumour Histopathology Reports: Royal College of Pathologists, April 2000.
11. Bostwick D. Natural history of early cancer. *J Cellul Biochem* 1992; **161**(suppl): 31–8.
12. Orozco R E, Martin A A, Murphy W M. Carcinoma in-situ of the urinary bladder. *Cancer* 1994; **74**: 115–22.
13. Parkin D M, Ferlay J, Hamdi-Cherif M *et al. Cancer in Africa: Epidemiology and Prevention.* IARC Scientific Publication No. 153. Lyon: IARC Press, 2003.
14. Lynch C F, Cohen M B. Urinary System. *Cancer* 1995; **75**: 316–29.

2

Clinical features of bladder cancer

Sarb Sandhu and Alan Thompson

Introduction

The etiology of bladder cancer is multifactorial, with chemical carcinogens, viruses, bacteria and other inducing agents causing aberrations in DNA. This can lead to the induction of oncogenes, the negation of suppressor genes and the failure of DNA repair mechanisms. This, coupled with inherited, acquired or anatomic factors, will determine whether individuals, when exposed to identical mutagens, will go on to develop bladder cancer or not. Once urothelial malignancy has developed, the entire urothelium can be affected, from the renal pelvis to the urethra; this field change coupled with the ability of transitional cell carcinoma to implant makes surveillance of the whole urinary tract essential.

Epidemiology

Bladder cancer has a male preponderance, with an incidence in males of 30 per 100 000 compared to 10 per 100 000 in females. There has been an increase in the incidence of bladder cancer in both sexes. In view of the negligible rates of detection of incidental bladder cancer during autopsy studies, this increase is unlikely to be because of better detection of indolent disease.

The mortality rate for bladder cancer is twice as high in men (11 per 100 000) as in women (5.7 per 100 000). The incidence of bladder cancer increases with age, with a peak between 80 and 84 years of age. Elderly patients with this disease have a higher mortality. This may be related to the advanced stage of the disease at presentation, coupled with possibly the biologic response of the elderly to this disease [1]. Aggressive treatment of this disease has been advocated in appropriate elderly patients with good response.

Carcinoma of the Bladder, ed. David MacVicar. Published by Cambridge University Press. © Cambridge University Press 2008.

Etiology

Environmental, chemical and anatomical predisposition

The most common causes of bladder cancer are cancer-inducing chemicals, such as aromatic amines (found in paints, plastics, dyes and diesel exhaust fumes).

Smoking increases the risk of bladder cancer, and this is directly related to the number of pack years. The exact agent in cigarette smoke responsible for bladder cancer is not known. However, acetylation of chemicals is a common pathway for inactivating toxic substances and it is known that slow acetylators have a reduced ability to inactivate these agents, and therefore, slow acetylation predisposes to the development of bladder cancer [2].

Some authorities have implicated coffee and tea drinking in the development of bladder cancer, but this is at present contentious. Abuse of the paracetamol derivative phenacetin has been associated with the development of transitional cell carcinoma throughout the urinary tract [3]. Animal studies using high doses of artificial sweeteners have caused bladder cancer in rodents though not in primates [4].

Other common predisposing factors include pelvic irradiation and cyclophosphamide. A relatively new agent involved in the development of urothelial malignancy is *Aristolochia fangchi* (a chinese herb) used in dieting. This leads to the development of a nephropathy and subsequently transitional cell carcinoma, which can affect the entire urinary tract [5]. Several groups are currently studying the role of viral agents, such as human paipilloma virus (HPV), which may have a role in causation of urothelial malignancy in immuno-compromised patients.

The majority (90%) of bladder cancer is transitional cell carcinoma. Other types of bladder cancer are less common. Infection with *Schistosoma haematobium* can lead to bilharzial squamous cell carcinoma, which is usually exophytic, nodular and fungating. Patients with this disease have a relatively low risk of lymph node and distant metastases. Non-bilharzial squamous cell epithelium (SCC) is usually a response to chronic urothelial irritation with stones, catheters or infections. This can lead to treatment dilemmas in this group of patients, who can be incapacitated and infirm, and so difficult to treat effectively.

Adenocarcinoma of the bladder can arise from three sources: the urachal remnant, primary vesical disease (often in association with bladder extrophy) or hematogenous metastases.

The bladder can also be the site of cancer invading directly from other organs in the pelvis, which may be any of a variety of cell types. Some of these, such as cervical cancer, may have independent etiological factors.

Genetic predisposition

The carcinogens implicated in bladder cancer lead to genetic mutations through a number of pathways including the activation of oncogenes, the inactivation of tumor suppressor genes, and over-expression of normal genes. Reports suggest that in as many as 50% of cases the p21 ras oncogene is activated, leading to aberrant activation of the membrane GTPase, thereby causing nuclear proliferation and de-differentiation. Other oncogenes linked to bladder cancer are Erb-2, EGFR, MDM2, C-MYC and CCND1 [6].

An alternative pathway for the development of malignancy is the inactivation of tumor suppressor genes. The p53 tumor suppressor gene characterized by Lane [7] is responsible for chaperoning cells with genetic aberrations toward apoptosis. The p53 gene is the most frequently altered gene in human cancer, and loss of the wild-type p53 results in the production of a protein with a much longer half-life. The presence of this aberrant protein and the loss of the native protein results in the loss of apoptosis and so aberrant cells may become "immortal." In common with many other tumors, bladder cancers with p53 abnormalities behave in a much more aggressive manner than those without.

Aberration in the retinoblastoma gene (13q) and its regulator proteins – p21, p27/KIP1, p16, coded on the neighbouring chromosome 9p – results in loss of control in the cell cycle. Abnormal expression of the retinoblastoma gene or its products also results in aggressive tumors. Other tumor suppressor genes associated with bladder cancer are PTEN, STK15, FHIT, FEZ1/LZTS1 and bc10 [6].

Over-expression of the endothelial growth factor (EGF) receptor leads to cell growth and increased cell motility, which is necessary for invasion and metastasis and essential for the development of malignancy.

A combination of these molecular markers may be helpful in predicting prognosis. In retrospective studies, the levels and mutational status of p53, p21 and the retinoblastoma gene were able to predict the recurrence and five-year survival rates in patients with muscle invasive bladder cancer [8].

Trends in the management of bladder cancer in the UK

In the United Kingdom, there has been a concerted effort to detect bladder cancer at an early clinicopathological stage. Patients of any age with frank hematuria, and those above 50 years of age with microscopic hematuria, can be referred to fast-track one-stop hematuria clinics. Approximately 25% of patients with frank hematuria, and 3.7% of patients with microscopic hematuria prove to have urological malignancy [9]. Patients are seen in fast-track hematuria clinics within two weeks of referral. Patients are assessed with a clinical history, urine cytology, upper tract imaging and a flexible cystoscopy to diagnose urothelial malignancy. There does appear to be a difference in the detection rates of urological malignancy in patients with dipstick hematuria who are diagnosed and investigated in Primary Care clinics compared to those that Primary Care physicians have referred to hospital hematuria clinics [10].

It is hoped that this will lead to an improvement in outcomes in patients with bladder cancer. Screening studies have demonstrated a possible stage shift at diagnosis, which may lead to improved outcomes. The average district general hospital serving 500 000 patients will diagnose 50 new patients with bladder cancer per year. The overall survival of patients with bladder cancer in the United Kingdom is similar to the European average.

At the time of writing, best practice in the United Kingdom is that all patients with newly diagnosed bladder cancer and aggressive bladder cancer should be discussed by a multidisciplinary team (MDT) that comprises urological surgeons, oncologists, histopathologists, radiologists and support professionals. The MDT undertakes formal review of diagnosis and staging in a forum which will allow the formulation of the optimum treatment strategy for each patient.

Patients with superficial disease are treated locally in district general hospital cancer units, but if the disease is muscle invasive, the patients are usually referred to cancer center. Of those patients who are shown to have muscle invasive disease, in a majority (possibly up to 90%) it is demonstrated at the time of first diagnosis. Some urologists consider the two diseases as distinct, with different outcomes and treatment options, only linked by the common organ of origin. It is hoped that this system of rapid referral to cancer center will minimize delays in treatment, allowing expertise to develop in center treating large numbers of patients with the disease, and improve outcomes.

Clinical presentation and initial management

The majority of patients with bladder cancer present with painless hematuria. This may be frank, microscopic or dipstick. Other less common presentations of bladder cancer are bladder irritability, frequency, urgency and flank pain (associated with ureteric obstruction). A pelvic mass associated with symptoms of longstanding bladder outflow obstruction is occasionally seen at presentation and indicates a poor prognosis, as does leg edema associated with nodal involvement.

Screening of patients with hematuria includes the classic triad of urine cytology, upper tract imaging and cystoscopy. High-grade malignant urothelial cancer (CIS and G3 urothelial cancer) has tumor cells with low cohesive potential which shed easily, and therefore can be detected in voided samples. The detection rates can be improved by using samples from bladder washings. Urine cytology alone, however, is not a cost-effective method of screening the general population for bladder cancer due to its limited usefulness in low grade and low stage tumors.

Imaging (either intravenous urography (IVU) or ultrasound (US), or both) is useful for diagnosing upper tract causes of hematuria or ureteric obstruction (see Chapter 3). The presence of hydronephrosis is an adverse prognostic factor in patients with muscle invasive disease [11].

Cystoscopy in fast-track clinics is usually carried out with a flexible cystoscope with local anesthetic. Ninety-nine percent of all bladder cancers can be diagnosed with cystoscopy. Flexible cystoscopy allows visualization of the bladder mucosa; biopsy of suspicious areas; and in patients with a known history of bladder cancer, treatment of small-volume disease by means of laser ablation of low-grade superficial tumors. Rigid cystoscopy is carried out under general or regional anesthesia. This is usually reserved for a bladder lesion previously detected on imaging or if there is a high index of suspicion that biopsies or resection of an extensive tumor will be required.

Blue-light cystoscopy involves the pre-installation of protoporhyrin precursor delta-5-amino-levulonic acid. Tumor cells preferentially retain this fluorescing agent. When blue-light cystoscopy is carried out, areas of tumor fluoresce, leading to increased sensitivity in detecting urothelial bladder carcinoma. The role for this technology is probably restricted to patients who have persistently positive cytology in the absence of obvious bladder tumor on visualization of the urothelium of both the upper and lower tracts.

Newer urinary molecular markers are being investigated. These include nuclear matrix protein 22, fibrin-degradation products, Quanticyt and Immunocyt. These tests have a high sensitivity and low specificity; therefore a large number of false positive tests can be generated. The role of these tests in the management of bladder cancer in clinical practice has yet to be defined.

Effect of staging and grading of bladder cancer on initial management

The bladder is covered by urothelial cells; these are multilayered and are attached to a basement membrane. The urothelial basement membrane is separated from the detrusor muscle of the bladder by the lamina propria. The lamina propria consists of loose connective tissue, inflammatory cells, vessels and strands of muscularis mucosae.

The management of bladder cancer is largely dependent upon whether the tumor invades the detrusor muscle. This is determined by resection specimens obtained at transurethral resection of bladder tumors and the obligatory examination under anesthetic. If the tumor is superficial and does not invade the lamina propria, it is stage pTa, if it invades the lamina propria then the tumor is stage pT1. Thirty percent of patients who demonstrate invasion of lamina propria (T1) will progress to muscle invasive disease (T2). T3 tumor invades perivesical tissue, and T4 invades adjacent organs. The treatment of superficial tumors principally involves endoscopic resection or fugaration. Intravesical agents are used to try to reduce the risk of recurrence or progression. Muscle invasive tumors require more radical treatments such as the total removal of the bladder, with some form of urinary diversion, or the use of radiotherapy.

The grade of the tumor is determined by the cytological appearance. High-stage disease is often accompanied by high-grade disease. The WHO 1973 grading system has been validated in many studies. Using this system, bladder carcinoma is graded from G1 to G3. In 2004 a new grading system was proposed. This divided urothelial carcinoma into low and high grade, eliminating the intermediate group, and also differentiated between urothelial carcinoma and papillary urothelial neoplasms of low malignant potential (PUNLMP), which are lesions with benign cytological appearance and have a negligible risk of progression, but can recur. The 2004 grading system has not yet been fully validated and in some units the older system is still preferred (see Chapter 1).

Carcinoma *in situ* (CIS) deserves particular mention. Uniquely in bladder cancer, the presence of an *in situ* component of the disease is an adverse prognostic feature. Carcinoma *in situ* presents with irritative symptoms. On visual cystoscopic inspection of the bladder, CIS can be undetectable, or classically appear as red velvety patches. Histological examination reveals severe cytological atypia. A high proportion of such patients will subsequently develop invasive bladder cancer and even succumb to their disease. Intravesical Bacille Calmette–Guérin (BCG) is the only accepted treatment for CIS. The presence of CIS resistant to BCG is an indication for radical cystectomy.

Patients with superficial low-grade disease (G1–2 pTa/pT1) can be treated with endoscopic resection, a single intravesical installation of mitomycin and surveillance. If a patient has frequent recurrences, the use of a six-week course of once-weekly intravesical mitomycin or BCG is recommended. The follow-up schedule is discussed in Chapter 9. Patients with high-grade superficial disease (G3pTa) are initially treated with endoscopic resection, intravesical mitomycin and surveillance. The threshold for adding a six-week course of BCG to these patients' regimen is lower. In patients with high-grade disease, BCG is usually preferred to mitomycin. Rigorous surveillance is carried out, and approximately 30% of patients with high-grade superficial disease will progress to muscle invasive disease, particularly if concomitant CIS is present.

Patients with muscle invasive organ-confined disease will usually be staged with cross-sectional imaging of abdomen and pelvis, and with increasing frequency the chest to exclude metastasis (see Chapter 4). If the disease is organ confined, the patients need to be treated with radical surgery (cystectomy) or radical radiotherapy with curative intent. There are many factors that will influence the choice of radical treatment for muscle invasive bladder cancer. Patients' age and comorbidity will influence the choice of treatment. Traditionally, surgical removal has been seen as the gold standard of treatment for such patients. With the advent of improved chemotherapy and radiotherapy techniques, however, more patients are choosing these modalities in an attempt at organ preservation. The volume and extent of disease will also influence the choice of treatment, e.g. large volume disease, urethral disease and disease causing hydronephrosis are best served by surgery. Adjuvant chemotherapy following surgery is increasingly being accepted as the norm in the management of muscle invasive bladder cancer (see Chapter 8).

Patients with disease that is not confined to the bladder at the time of diagnosis require bespoke treatment, as befits their needs. This can include palliative chemotherapy, radiotherapy or symptom control.

Conclusion

Bladder cancer has a multifocal etiology and is increasing in incidence. Hematuria is the presenting symptom in up to 90% of patients with bladder cancer, while the chance of finding a tumor in a patient with frank hematuria is approximately 25%. The majority of bladder cancers will be diagnosed by cystoscopy and resection. At diagnosis, approximately 70% of tumors will be superficial and low grade in nature. Of these, approximately 85% will remain superficial in nature although many are likely to recur. Treatment schedules and consequent follow-up schedules are based not only on the stage and grade at the time of diagnosis but also on the likelihood of recurrence and progression.

REFERENCES

1. Nielsen M E, Shariat S F, Karakiewicz P I. *et al.* for the Bladder Cancer Research Consortium (BCRC). Advanced age is associated with poorer bladder cancer-specific survival in patients treated with radical cystectomy. *Eur Urol* 2007; **51**: 699–708.
2. Marcus P M, Hayes R B, Vineis P *et al.* Cigarette smoking, N-acetyltransferase 2 acetylation status, and bladder cancer risk: a case-series meta-analysis of a gene-environment interaction. *Cancer Epidemiol Biomarkers Prev* 2000; **9**: 461–7.
3. Piper J M, Tonascia J, Matanoski G M. Heavy phenacetin use and bladder cancer in women aged 20 to 49 years. *N Engl J Med* 1985; **313**: 292–5.
4. Takayama S, Sieber S M, Adamson R H *et al.* Long-term feeding of sodium saccharin to nonhuman primates: implications for urinary tract cancer. *J Natl Cancer Inst* 1998; **90**: 19–25.
5. Nortier J L, Martinez M C, Schmeiser H H *et al.* Urothelial carcinoma associated with the use of a Chinese herb (Aristolochia fangchi). *N Engl J Med* 2000; **342**: 1686–92.
6. Baffa R, Letko J, McClung C *et al.* Molecular genetics of bladder cancer: targets for diagnosis and therapy. *J Exp Clin Cancer Res* 2006; **25**: 145–60.
7. Lane D P. Cancer. p53, guardian of the genome. *Nature* 1992; **358**: 15–16.
8. Chatterjee S J, Datar R, Youssefzadeh D *et al.* Combined effects of p53, p21, and pRb expression in the progression of bladder transitional cell carcinoma. *J Clin Oncol* 2004; **22**: 1007–13.
9. Alishahi S, Byrne D, Goodman C M, Baxby K. Haematuria investigation based on a standard protocol: emphasis on the diagnosis of urological malignancy. *J R Coll Surg Edinb* 2002; **47**: 422–7.
10. National Institute for Clinical Excellence (NICE). Guidance on Cancer Services: Improving Outcomes in Urological Cancers. 2002: 12.
11. Bartsch G C, Kuefer R, Gschwend J E *et al.* Hydronephrosis as a prognostic marker in bladder cancer in a cystectomy-only series. *Eur Urol* 2007; **51**: 690–8.

3

Imaging in the diagnosis of bladder cancer

Sarah Williams and Aslam Sohaib

Introduction

The diagnosis of bladder cancer is histopathological and biopsy material is readily obtained at cystoscopy. Imaging does, however, have a number of roles complementing cystoscopy in evaluating the bladder for the detection and characterization of any bladder lesion and also in evaluating the upper tracts. In this chapter we review imaging techniques and the role of imaging in the diagnosis of bladder cancer.

Clinical presentation and management

Bladder cancer may be diagnosed in a variety of clinical scenarios. The commonest presenting symptom is painless macroscopic hematuria. Lower urinary tract symptoms such as dysuria, urgency or frequency are also common. Occasionally, the diagnosis may be made incidentally on imaging for an unrelated problem or it may be that metastatic disease (see Chapter 5) precipitates the initial clinical presentation of bladder cancer, e.g., cachexia or pain from bone metastasis, but this is very unusual.

Hematuria

Hematuria is a common urological symptom with a wide range of causes from pre-renal disorders such as coagulation dysfunction to renal and bladder causes. Painless macroscopic hematuria should be assumed to be secondary to a bladder tumor unless proven otherwise as over 80% of patients with bladder cancer present in this way [1]. Between the ages of 40 and 49 years, 16% of men with macroscopic

Carcinoma of the Bladder, ed. David MacVicar. Published by Cambridge University Press. © Cambridge University Press 2008.

hematuria have a urological cancer and in men between 50 and 59 years of age, 20% [2]. The incidence of bladder cancer is much lower in patients with microscopic hematuria, although it increases in patients over 50 years of age [3].

A range of evidence-based protocols have been suggested for the investigation of both micro- and macroscopic hematuria [4,5]. Recently, imaging of the upper tracts has moved from excretory urography to cross-sectional imaging such as computed tomography (CT), ultrasonography or magnetic resonance imaging (MRI). Cystoscopy and biopsy are, however, the standard for bladder evaluation, particularly for early stage disease, with imaging of more use in staging, complete evaluation of the uroepithelial tract and follow-up.

The American Urological Association guidelines require urological work-up for the investigation of patients with asymptomatic microscopic hematuria who have no evidence of primary renal disease and in whom benign causes have been excluded. Upper tract imaging evaluation is recommended with CT or excretory urography and bladder evaluation with cystoscopy [4].

One-stop clinics for the evaluation of patients with hematuria have been developing over the last 10–15 years. An example of the format would be that initially patients are invited for a consultation that includes taking a clinical history and performing a relevant physical examination. A flexible cystoscopy is carried out on all patients during the first visit. Other investigations include a repeat urine analysis, urine culture and cytology. Following this, the choice of upper tract imaging modality depends on the results of cystoscopy. Patients with bladder tumors are referred for urgent intravenous urogram to identify any upper tract transitional cell carcinoma (TCC) prior to transurethral resection. Otherwise, upper tract imaging comprises a radiograph of the kidney-ureter-bladder (KUB) and a renal ultrasound scan.

Diagnostic evaluation of bladder tumors

Cystoscopy

Performing cystoscopy and biopsy is the standard method for the diagnosis of bladder cancer. It is also used for surveillance of patients at risk of developing invasive bladder cancer. Cystoscopic evaluation allows assessment of the bladder mucosa, in particular regions of the vesical trigone with the ureteric orifices and the internal urethral orifice. Direct inspection also permits visualization of color change in the mucosa.

One-stop or fast-track hematuria clinics use flexible cystoscopes that require local anesthesia. Flexiscope is a fiber optic instrument that can bend easily and has a maneuverable tip that makes it easy to pass along the curves of the urethra. It is less traumatic and less painful than a rigid scope and is often successful after failure of rigid cystoscopy [6].

Rigid cystoscopy is carried out under general or regional anesthesia and uses a solid straight telescope. It is viewed as the gold standard in diagnosis of bladder lesions. It has a higher failure rate than flexible cystoscopes, in addition to more bleeding and problems with small volume bladders.

Fluorescence cystoscopy with pre-instillation of hexaminolevulinate (HAL) allows visualization of tumor cells as they preferentially retain the fluorescing agent. Fluorescence cystoscopy is superior to standard white light cystoscopy for detecting bladder carcinoma [7]. Its clinical application probably lies in the investigation of patients with positive cytology but no lesion seen on direct visualization.

Cystoscopic techniques do have limitations. It can be difficult to assess the bladder in patients with gross hematuria and the cystoscope is unable to assess the intraluminal component of a diverticulum for tumors. There are some patients in whom cystoscopy is contraindicated, such as in patients with bacteriuria, acute cystitis, urethritis, prostatitis, obstructive prostatic hypertrophy and stricture or rupture of the urethra. Cystoscopy is an invasive procedure that is uncomfortable and has associated risks such as infection, perforation, scarring and strictures.

Urine cytology

Urine cytology is an important non-invasive technique for diagnosis of urinary tract neoplasia. Voided urine cytology is a Pap smear of cells lining the urinary tract that have fallen off into the urine. This can detect malignant and premalignant cells. If the urinary cytology is positive, then transitional cell carcinoma of the urothelium is almost certainly present in the upper tracts or bladder. Cytological examinations may be negative in up to half of the patients with bladder cancer; thus, a negative study does not rule out bladder cancer [8].

Excretory urography

Excretory urography (intravenous urography) involves the injection of an iodinated intravenous contrast medium. Subsequent radiographs are taken sequentially to demonstrate the excretion of contrast into the kidneys, collecting systems, ureters and bladder. The primary bladder tumor may appear as a small-capacity thick-walled bladder or a focal mass within the bladder, which appears as a filling defect. If the tumor is multifocal, as occurs in 30% of patients, lesions may also be identified in the ureters or in the pelvicalyceal (PC) system. These lesions may appear as filling defects in the PC system or ureters, as distortion of the PC systems or as strictures along the course of the ureters. Tumor may cause obstruction proximally and dilatation of the renal collecting system. The main limitation of excretory urography is that superficial or small tumors may not be identified, and if a tumor is identified there is no indication of the degree of invasion.

Retrograde studies

Retrograde studies are used to image the upper urinary tract. This involves the cannulation of the ureter and instillation of contrast medium up the ureters and is done at the time of cystoscopy. Retrograde studies are used when other imaging techniques have not completely visualized the upper tracts or if urine cytology is suspicious or positive for malignancy in the absence of a tumor in the bladder at cystoscopy.

Ultrasound

Ultrasound is a useful technique for demonstrating a bladder tumor if it is larger than 0.5 cm, although tumors in the dome of the bladder or at the neck can be difficult to visualize [9]. They have the appearances of a papillary hypoechoic mass, or the focal area of the bladder wall thickening appears plaque-like. They appear vascular on color Doppler imaging, which helps differentiate tumor from clot. If there is calcification or fibrosis, there will be areas of increased echogenicity. Ultrasound is limited in that it is not good at evaluating the depth of tumor although surrounding adenopathy can be assessed. Three-dimensional ultrasound has been assessed and initial studies demonstrate that it is more accurate than standard 2D ultrasound, and therefore may become useful for routine evaluation of the bladder in the future [10].

Radionuclide imaging

Radionuclide imaging does not have a role in the diagnosis of bladder tumors as most of the tracer is excreted through the urine. Positron emission tomography

(PET) with F-18FDG is of limited value for detection of bladder cancer because of the urinary excretion of the tracer. Other tracers have been assessed and the primary tumor can be visualized with 11C-methionine but there is no evidence that this improves detection and it should not be routinely used [11].

Computed tomography

Computed tomography (CT) is a frequently used primary imaging modality for bladder cancer (Figs. 3.1, 3.2a and 3.3). Ideally, the bladder should be distended to increase the sensitivity for detecting a lesion and this allows more accurate staging. The patient should be scanned with intravenous contrast in the nephrographic phase (100–120 secs) before the contrast reaches the bladder so the enhancing

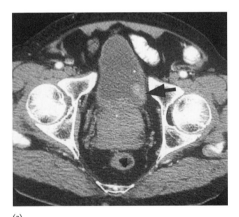

(a)

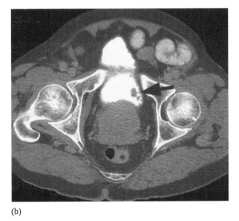

(b)

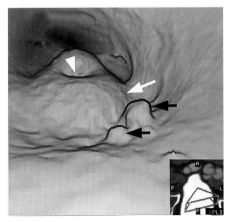

(c)

Figure 3.1 Transitional cell carcinoma of the bladder. Axial contrast-enhanced CT: (a) arterial phase image demonstrates the early enhancement of the polypoidal tumor (arrow); (b) delayed imaging with contrast within the bladder outlining the intraluminal growth (arrow). (c) Virtual cystoscopy reconstructed images show two polypoidal growths (black arrows) on the bladder wall. *Note*: Behind the polypoidal growths is the indentation from an enlarged prostate (white arrow) with the urethral orifice (white arrowhead) in the middle.

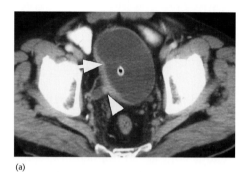

(a)

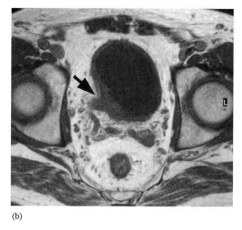

(b)

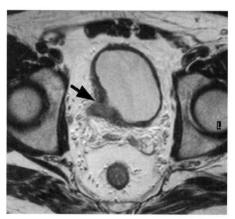

(c)

Figure 3.2 Transitional cell carcinoma of the bladder involving the distal right ureter. (a) Axial contrast-enhanced CT shows an enhancing soft tissue mass (white arrow) involving the right bladder wall, with a component (white arrowhead) seen to extend into the distal right ureter, which is dilated above this level. Axial (b) T1-weighted and (c) T2-weighted MR images show a soft tissue lesion extending into the lumen of the bladder and the right ureter (black arrows).

tumor can be seen against the low attenuation urine [12]. If there is some delay, a ureteral jet can mimic or obscure a malignant lesion. Computed tomography imaging will demonstrate an intraluminal papillary or nodular mass or focal wall thickening. These lesions demonstrate early and intense enhancement when compared to surrounding normal bladder (Figs. 3.1a and 3.2a). The lesions may contain nodular or surface calcification.

Axial CT images were known to be poor at demonstrating the base and dome of the bladder but this is no longer such an important issue with multidetector CT and multiplanar reformatting of images (Fig. 3.3). The limitation of CT is in its detection of small bladder cancers. There are many confounding factors that make the assessment of the bladder difficult including recent biopsy or inflammation, which can

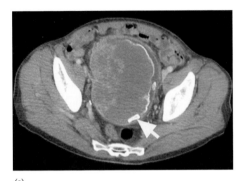

(a)

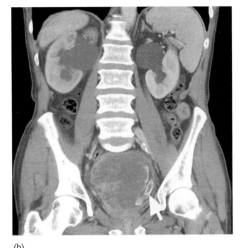

(b)

Figure 3.3 Squamous cell carcinoma of the
bladder. Contrast-enhanced CT with (a) axial,
(b) coronal and (c) paracoronal reformatted images
of the abdomen and pelvis. A large heterogenous
tumor is seen arising from the right lateral bladder
wall and occupying most of the bladder. The tumor
shows surface calcification (arrows) and is causing
bilateral hydronephrosis. Cystectomy was
performed and histology showed this to be pT1b
poorly differentiated squamous cell carcinoma.

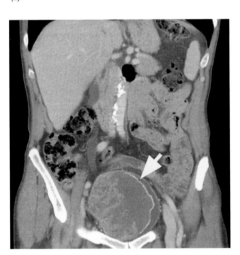

(c)

mimic a cancer. Radiation leading to fibrosis can also lead to bladder wall thickening
(and stranding of the pelvic fat), as can chemotherapy (systemic cyclophosphamide
and ifosfamide or intravesical Bacillus Calmette–Guérin or formalin).

Computed tomography urography

The technique CT urography (CTU) refers to images obtained of the bladder and
renal tract when contrast media has reached the renal collecting system and

bladder, i.e. in the urographic phase. This method has the advantage over conventional CT of the abdomen and pelvis in that it is tailored to visualize the urinary tract only. Protocols of CTU usually incorporate precontrast images as well as images in the nephrographic phase of enhancement, using a time delay of approximately 100–120 seconds from commencement of injection. These techniques therefore allow for detailed assessment of the renal parenchyma as well as the collecting systems, thereby allowing the detection of coexisting urothelial tumors. It is a quicker examination than standard excretory urography and has been demonstrated to have a greater accuracy [13]. In some centers, CTU has replaced the combination of ultrasound and excretory urography in the assessment of hematuria. Mass lesions of the bladder and renal tract as well as pelvicalyceal abnormality can all be evaluated.

There are a large range of CTU protocols, and to date studies have not shown a significant advantage of any particular protocol. An example of a 3-phase protocol used at our institution begins with intravenous hydration with 250 ml of normal saline 10–15 minutes before the scan commences. No oral contrast is given. Images are then acquired as thin-section precontrast axial scans through the urinary tract. Then, 150 ml of intravenous iodinated contrast is administered and thin-section acquisition is made from the top of the kidneys to the pubic symphysis at 100 seconds after contrast (nephrographic phase) and then at 7½ minutes (excretory phase) [14]. Axial reconstructions and orthogonal plane reformats are then produced for interpretation and archiving.

Magnetic resonance imaging (MRI)

The high soft tissue contrast resolution of MRI has advantages over CT studies as it may allow distinction of bladder wall layers, which is useful in staging bladder tumors (see Chapter 4). However, this soft tissue resolution can also assist in the detection of bladder tumors, along with direct multiplanar imaging, which is useful in detecting lesions in the dome or base of the bladder. Bladder tumors are typically of intermediate signal intensity on T1- and T2-weighted sequences, with urine within the lumen returning low signal intensity on T1-weighted images but high signal intensity on T2-weighted sequences (Figs. 3.2b,c and 3.4). These sequences can be supplemented with fast, dynamic, contrast-enhanced T1-weighted imaging. This will demonstrate the tumor, which is seen to enhance earlier than the adjacent bladder wall. The reported detection accuracy of MRI in the literature is in the region of 70–90% [15,16]. Dynamic gadolinium-enhanced MRI appears to result in

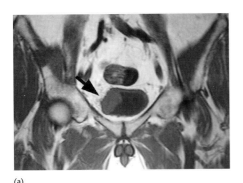
(a)

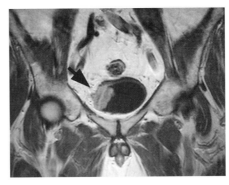
(b)

Figure 3.4 Transitional cell carcinoma of the bladder. Coronal T1-weighted (a) before and (b) after intravenous gadolinium and (c) axial T2-weighted images show a polypoidal enhancing soft tissue mass with extension through the bladder wall (arrow).

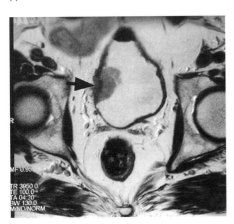
(c)

an increased detection rate [16]. Cancer detection rate is similar for both CT and MRI despite the improved soft tissue resolution of MRI, although the staging is more accurate with MRI [15].

Magnetic resonance urography

Urographic images can be obtained on MRI using two different techniques known as static and dynamic [17]. "Static" urographic images are acquired without using injection of intravenous gadolinium, and rely on contrast from static fluid by using a very heavily T2-weighted sequence [18]. Alternatively, "dynamic" images can be acquired in the excretory delayed phase following the administration of intravenous gadolinium in a similar manner to CT urography although this technique often requires a diuretic to allow for optimal opacification of the collecting systems [19]. Both MR urographic techniques in combination with standard MRI permit a comprehensive examination of entire urinary tract.

Virtual cystoscopy

Recent developments in imaging technologies have led to the various forms of virtual reality imaging. Acquisition of 3D imaging dataset and the application of volume/ surface rendering algorithms allow for generation of virtual cystoscopic images. CT virtual cystoscopy (CT VC) is emerging as a promising diagnostic tool. Early proto- cols involved filling the bladder with air or carbon dioxide (pneumocystoscopy) or iodinated contrast medium [20,21]. However, these techniques have the disadvantage of requiring urethral catheterization, with the associated contraindications and risks.

More recently, CT VC images have been obtained following injection of intra- venous contrast media and acquiring delayed images when the bladder feels full and has filled with contrast medium (this is usually at approximately 90–140 min) (Fig. 3.1). Prior to this delayed scan, the patient is rolled on the couch several times to mix urine with the contrast in the bladder. This technique is safer and more comfortable than catheterizing the patient and instilling contrast medium directly; however, it does carry the risk of contrast-induced nephrotoxicity or contrast reaction [21] .

The sensitivity of CT VC for detecting bladder tumors is reported to be over 90% [22,23]. However, for small lesions and sessile tumors the sensitivity is reduced, although recent papers have reported detection rates of up to 88% for lesions less than 5 mm [24]. Viewing images with VC has been shown to be better than multiplanar reformatted images as it is superior at detecting superficial lesions because it assesses the bladder mucosa [25]. Color mapping of the entire thickness of the bladder wall has also been used. This improves the sensitivity of detection of small or flat and sessile lesions [26,27].

In conjunction with the development of CT VC there has been the development of MR virtual cystoscopy (MR VC). It has advantages similar to that of CT VC. However, with MR VC the procedure can be conducted without external bladder filling and no intravenous contrast is required. For MR virtual cystoscopy, the patient is only required to have a distended bladder and 3D T2-weighted turbo spin echo images are acquired in the coronal plane. A variety of other imaging sequences have been described [28].

Studies evaluating MR VC have shown a detection rate of 100% for tumors greater than 1 cm, but for lesions less than 1 cm the rate reduced to 70% [29]. As with CT

VC, the difficulties that arose were in detection of flat bladder tumors that gave minimal elevation of the bladder surface. It was, however, noted that these tend to be histologically superficial tumors. With MR VC, it is difficult to differentiate between small tumors and inflammatory swelling of the mucosa, especially if the bladder is underfilled. It does, however, have the advantage over conventional and CT virtual cystoscopy in that it is good in imaging patients with gross hematuria, as this does not affect the sensitivity of MR imaging. The other advantage shared by CT and MR VC over the conventional cystoscopic method is that the anterior bladder wall and bladder diverticulae are easier to scrutinize.

Limitations of MR VC include any contraindications to MR imaging as well as artifact encountered from metal prostheses. Further artifacts that may arise include wrap-around, striping and motion artifacts from long echo times such as scanner vibration and detrusor contraction. Another factor to be considered is the scanning time and associated cost, and the processing and evaluation time, which is between 15 and 40 minutes.

Virtual cystoscopy whether by CT or MR has the advantage that it can be utilized in patients in whom conventional cystoscopy is contraindicated or difficult. Positive findings at VC can be very helpful in managing such patients. However, limitations of the techniques must be appreciated when the findings at VC are negative, i.e. sessile lesion and carcinoma *in situ*. The findings at VC would be used in conjunction with imaging of the upper tracts, urine cytology and clinical assessment. The disadvantage of all virtual techniques is that although a diagnosis and staging can be reached, a tissue sample for histological diagnosis is not obtained. Virtual cystoscopy is also limited in patients who have had prior bladder surgery or radiotherapy as this distorts the bladder contour and interpretation of the anatomy becomes difficult.

Imaging characteristics of histological subtypes

Although all of the above techniques may detect thickening of the bladder wall, they cannot give a definitive pathological diagnosis. In addition to malignant neoplasms, there are many other causes of bladder wall thickening. These include benign neoplasms such as papillomas, hamartomas and leiomyomas. Other causes of focal bladder wall thickening or masses include hematomas, calculi, fungus balls, cystitis cystica, foreign bodies and endometriosis. There is overlap in the clinical and radiological findings of bladder tumors; however, some tumors do have individual features which can give a clue to the underlying histopathological diagnosis [30].

Transitional cell carcinoma

There are certain features that are common to TCC that can be identified on imaging, although none is entirely specific. The majority occur at the bladder base and approximately half will be larger than 2.5 cm at diagnosis. They may be papillary, sessile or nodular (Figs. 3.1, 3.2 and 3.4) and the pattern of growth correlates with the likelihood of invasion. Sessile lesions have a higher propensity to muscle invasion and are usually of higher grade than papillary lesions [31]. Most patients have a superficial papillary tumor at cystoscopy. Calcification is rare (5%) unlike other types of neoplasm such as adenocarcinoma (50% calcification). Approximately 30% of these tumors will be multicentric with synchronous and metachronous bladder and upper tract tumors. Upper tract tumors are more common if there are multicentric bladder lesions present and therefore the upper tracts must be scrutinized in these cases. Despite the above features, the differential diagnosis for these lesions seen on imaging must be considered. Papillary lesions may be papillomas or papillary urothelial neoplasm of low malignant potential (PUNLMP). Sessile lesions can be due to hyperplasia, atypia or carcinoma *in situ*.

Squamous cell carcinoma

Squamous cell carcinoma (SCC) accounts for less than 5% of bladder neoplasms in the West, although it is a major health problem in countries where schistosomiasis is endemic. Other risk factors for bladder SCC include stones, indwelling catheters or chronic infection. The imaging features of SCC are in some ways different to TCC. They usually consist of a single sessile enhancing mass or diffuse or focal bladder wall thickening most commonly around the trigone and lateral bladder wall. They can have surface calcification encrusting the tumor, which is most readily demonstrated on CT imaging (Fig. 3.3). Unlike TCC they rarely demonstrate pure intraluminal growth. This does mean that 80% demonstrate muscle invasion at diagnosis and extensive extravesical spread to other organs, and pelvic and abdominal wall invasion is frequently found. Despite this, only 1 in 10 patients will have metastases at diagnosis [32].

Adenocarcinoma

Adenocarcinoma accounts for less than 2% of bladder cancers and may be a primary or secondary tumor. Metastatic adenocarcinoma is the more common and is the commonest secondary to the bladder. Bladder involvement is often a late manifestation so signs of the primary or other metastases are already present. Direct invasion of the bladder occurs from primaries of the prostate, ovary, colon or rectum. Hematogenous spread occurs most commonly from the stomach, breast or lung. It is important to differentiate primary from metastatic bladder adenocarcinoma due to the difference in treatments.

Primary bladder adenocarcinoma can be nonurachal (66%) or urachal. Urachal adenocarcinoma is associated with bladder extrophy and persistent urachus, urothelial metaplasia from mucosal irritation, urinary diversions and pelvic lipomatosis. A quarter of urachal adenocarcinomas will have mucus in the urine.

On imaging, urachal adenocarcinoma appears as a large mixed solid and cystic lesion, with approximately 70% of the lesions demonstrating calcification, which is usually around the edge of the tumor and is patchy rather than continuous, unlike the surface calcification in SCC [33]. The bulk of the tumor is outside the bladder and extravesical spread is common. Because of mucin secretion from these tumors, they show high signal on T2-weighted MRI sequences. Urachal tumors commonly arise at the dome in the midline, with 10% identified along the course of the urachus. They are therefore seen as a midline infra-umbilical soft tissue mass with calcification. Sagittal imaging is therefore ideal to demonstrate these lesions. At diagnosis they are usually large (over 5 cm) and peritoneal metastases are common [33].

Non-urachal adenocarcinoma has different imaging characteristics, with 75% appearing as diffuse bladder wall thickening commonly at the bladder base and the majority demonstrating associated stranding of the perivesical fat (Figs. 3.5 and 3.6) [34]. These malignancies are frequently present

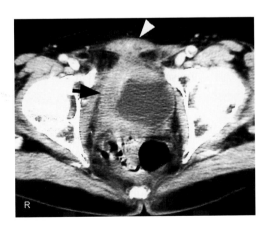

Figure 3.5 **Non-urachal adenocarcinoma of the bladder. Axial contrast-enhanced CT shows bladder wall thickening (arrow) with extravesical stranding and extension to the rectus abdominis muscle anteriorly (white arrowhead).**

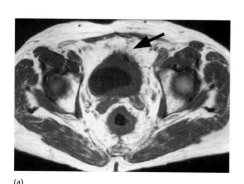 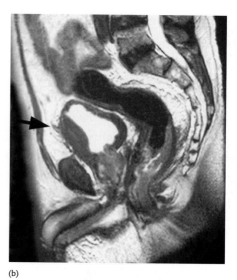

(a)   (b)

Figure 3.6   Non-urachal adenocarcinoma of the bladder. (a) Axial T1-weighted and (b) sagittal T2-weighted image shows circumferential bladder wall thickening of approximately three quarters of the bladder wall with extensive perivesical stranding (arrow).

with locally advanced disease, and a large proportion of patients have distant metastases. The peritoneum, lymph nodes, and lung are the most common sites [34].

Lymphoma

The bladder can be a site of primary lymphoma, or it may be involved by secondary lymphoma during the course of the disease [35]. Bladder involvement is almost invariably non-Hodgkin's lymphoma rather than Hodgkin's disease. The malignant clone of cells arises from lymphoid tissue within the bladder wall. The pattern of growth is analogous to that seen in other hollow viscera such as the gut. The wall thickens in a manner which becomes fusiform. Disease may become bulky by the time of presentation as lymphoma may remain submucosal in its early stages, with the result that hematuria is not pronounced. The mucosal surface at cystoscopy may remain intact, and deeper biopsy than normal may be necessary. Cross-sectional imaging can be helpful in these clinical circumstances in demonstrating a bulky mass with relatively few clinical symptoms (Fig. 3.7). Obstructive urinary symptoms and hydronephrosis occur late in bladder lymphoma, probably as a result of the tumor being relatively soft. Treatment is with chemotherapy, and the

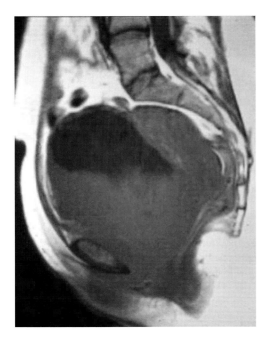

Figure 3.7 Lymphoma of the bladder. T1-weighted sagittal MRI in a female patient demonstrates gross thickening of the bladder wall at its base. Some urinary symptoms were present but these were longstanding and not severe. Biopsy demonstrated a primary bladder non-Hodgkin's lymphoma.

lymphoid neoplasm should usually respond favorably. The morphology of the bladder will return to close to normal, although some residual mural thickening may be observed.

Bladder involvement may also be seen as a result of metastatic lymphoma, but this is rare, and is usually seen in the clinical context of a high grade or aggressive lymphoma. The imaging features are similar to those observed with primary bladder lymphoma.

Other unusual tumors

There are a number of rare types of bladder tumor which include small cell carcinoma, neuroendocrine tumors such as carcinoid, leiomyoma, sarcoma, melanoma, neurofibroma and paraganglioma [36] (Fig. 3.8). Non-malignant lesions such as hemangiomas and endometriosis may mimic bladder cancer, but there may be some clues to an alternative diagnosis. For example, cyclical hematuria is the classical clinical presentation of endometriosis affecting the bladder. Magnetic resonance imaging may reveal subtle signal changes which suggest hemorrhage in association with endometriosis (Fig. 3.9) [37]. Primary melanoma may affect any mucosal surface, including the urothelium (Fig. 3.10). However, many of these

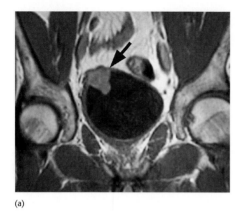

(a)

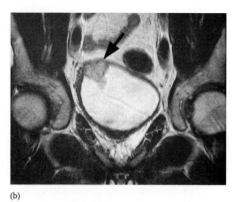

(b)

Figure 3.8 Bladder phaeochromocytoma. Coronal (a) T1-weighted images following intravenous gadolinium and (b) fast spin-echo T2-weighted images demonstrate a polypoidal lesion (arrow) in the dome of the bladder. The lesion enhances following intravenous gadolinium and is of increased signal intensity (but not as high as urine) on the T2-weighted images typical for a pheochromocytoma.

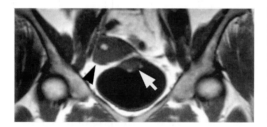

Figure 3.9 Endometriosis involving the bladder. Unenhanced T1-weighted coronal image of bladder. There is a mass on the dome of the bladder with some surface hemorrhage (arrow). Note also a mixed signal mass adjacent to the bladder (arrowhead), which represents forms of endometriosis on the pelvic peritoneum (reproduced with permission from Ref. [37]).

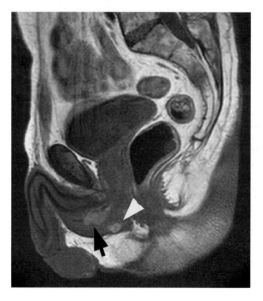

Figure 3.10 Melanoma. Mucosal lesion as presentation of primary melanoma of bladder. Gadolinium-enhanced T1-weighted sagittal image showing primary melanoma of the posterior urethra (arrow) with an intransit lesion (arrowhead).

rare tumors are diagnosed after cystoscopy and the biopsy result may prove to be a surprise.

When there is a history of pre-existing malignancy, metastatic disease should always be a consideration. Metastatic involvement from local pelvic tumors is usually associated with a mass lesion in the vicinity. Direct spread of prostatic carcinoma onto the bladder base may have imaging characteristics similar to that

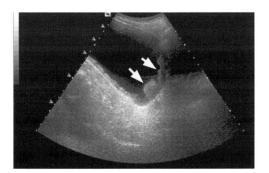

Figure 3.11 Prostatic carcinoma involving bladder. Sagittal ultrasound showing prostatic carcinoma invading bladder base (arrows).

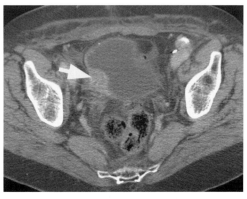

Figure 3.12 Recurrent ovarian carcinoma. CT shows a mass lesion (arrow) as a result of peritoneal recurrence invading the bladder wall.

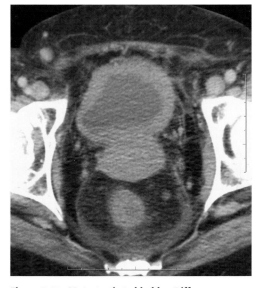

Figure 3.13 Metastastis to bladder. Diffuse thickening of bladder wall as a result of metastatic breast cancer. There was also diffuse involvement of the peritoneal cavity.

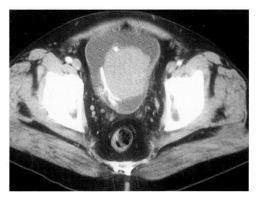

Figure 3.14 Metastasis to the bladder. Mass lesion in the bladder is a deposit of metastatic malignant melanoma.

of a bladder primary (Fig. 3.11). However, it is not unusual for ovarian carcinoma, following resection at hysterectomy and bilateral salpingo-oophorectomy, to recur over the surface of the bladder in the absence of bulk disease at the site of surgery (Fig. 3.12). Diffuse thickening of the bladder may be seen in the presence of peritoneal disease against the background of gastric or pancreatic malignancy. Peritoneal disease may also result from transcoelomic spread of tumors such as breast carcinoma (Fig. 3.13). Very rarely an intraluminal deposit may be seen in the bladder in the context of disseminated cancer, usually a result of an aggressive tumor such as sarcoma or melanoma (Fig. 3.14).

Conclusion

Imaging plays an important role in conjunction with cystoscopy and biopsy in the diagnosis of bladder cancer. Certain tumor types have characteristic features, such as multiplicity of TCC and mucin content of urachal adenocarcinoma. Histology is always necessary to establish tumor type even when typical imaging features are observed.

REFERENCES

1. Pashos C L, Botteman M F, Laskin B L, Redaelli A. Bladder cancer: epidemiology, diagnosis, and management. *Cancer Pract* 2002; **10**(6): 311–22.
2. Khadra M H, Pickard R S, Charlton M *et al.* A prospective analysis of 1,930 patients with hematuria to evaluate current diagnostic practice. *J Urol* 2000; **163**(2): 524–7.
3. Kirkali Z, Chan T, Manoharan M *et al.* Bladder cancer: epidemiology, staging and grading, and diagnosis. *Urology* 2005; **66**(6 suppl. 1): 4–34.
4. Grossfeld G D, Litwin M S, Wolf J S Jr., *et al.* Evaluation of asymptomatic microscopic hematuria in adults: the American Urological Association best practice policy – part II: patient evaluation, cytology, voided markers, imaging, cystoscopy, nephrology evaluation, and follow-up. *Urology* 2001; **57**(4): 604–10.
5. Fickenscher L. Evaluating adult hematuria. *Nurse Pract* 1999; **24**(9): 58–65.
6. Ambartsumian A M. The efficacy of rigid and flexible endoscopes in the diagnosis of bladder diseases. *Urol Nefrol (Mosk)* 1989; **1**: 51–3.
7. Witjes J A, Moonen P M, van der Heijden A G. Comparison of hexaminolevulinate based flexible and rigid fluorescence cystoscopy with rigid white light cystoscopy in bladder cancer: results of a prospective Phase II study. *Eur Urol* 2005; **47**(3): 319–22.

8. Badalament R A, Kimmel M, Gay H *et al*. The sensitivity of flow cytometry compared with conventional cytology in the detection of superficial bladder carcinoma. *Cancer* 1987; **59**(12): 2078–85.

9. Itzchak Y, Singer D, Fischelovitch Y. Ultrasonographic assessment of bladder tumors. I. Tumor detection. *J Urol* 1981; **126**(1): 31–3.

10. Mitterberger M, Pinggera G M, Neuwirt H *et al*. Three-dimensional ultrasonography of the urinary bladder: preliminary experience of assessment in patients with haematuria. *BJU Int* 2007; **99**(1): 111–16.

11. Hain S F. Positron emission tomography in uro-oncology. *Cancer Imaging* 2005; **5**(1): 1–7.

12. Kim J K, Park S Y, Ahn H J *et al*. Bladder cancer: analysis of multi-detector row helical CT enhancement pattern and accuracy in tumor detection and perivesical staging. *Radiology* 2004; **231**(3): 725–31.

13. Caoili E M, Cohan R H, Inampudi P *et al*. MDCT urography of upper tract urothelial neoplasms. *AJR Am J Roentgenol* 2005; **184**(6): 1873–81.

14. Caoili E M, Inampudi P, Cohan R H, Ellis J. Optimization of multi-detector row CT urography: effect of compression, saline administration, and prolongation of acquisition delay. *Radiology* 2005; **235**(1): 116–23.

15. Kim B, Semelka R C, Ascher S M *et al*. Bladder tumor staging: comparison of contrast-enhanced CT, T1- and T2-weighted MR imaging, dynamic gadolinium-enhanced imaging, and late gadolinium-enhanced imaging. *Radiology* 1994; **193**(1): 239–45.

16. Neuerburg J M, Bohndorf K, Sohn M *et al*. Staging of urinary bladder neoplasms with MR imaging: is Gd-DTPA helpful? *J Comput Assist Tomogr* 1991; **15**(5): 780–6.

17. Nolte-Ernsting C C, Adam G B, Gunther R W. MR urography: examination techniques and clinical applications. *Eur Radiol* 2001; **11**(3): 355–72.

18. Rothpearl A, Frager D, Subramanian A *et al*. MR urography: technique and application. *Radiology* 1995; **194**(1): 125–30.

19. Nolte-Ernsting C C, Bucker A, Adam G B *et al*. Gadolinium-enhanced excretory MR urography after low-dose diuretic injection: comparison with conventional excretory urography. *Radiology* 1998; **209**(1): 147–57.

20. Kishore T A, George G K, Bhat S. Virtual cystoscopy by intravesical instillation of dilute contrast medium: preliminary experience. *J Urol* 2006; **175**(3 Pt 1): 870–4.

21. Kawai N, Mimura T, Nagata D *et al*. Intravenous urography-virtual cystoscopy is a better preliminary examination than air virtual cystoscopy. *BJU Int* 2004; **94**(6): 832–6.

22. Arslan H, Ceylan K, Harman M *et al*. Virtual computed tomography cystoscopy in bladder pathologies. *Int Braz J Urol* 2006; **32**(2): 147–54; discussion 154.

23. Nambirajan T, Sohaib S A, Muller-Pollard C *et al*. Virtual cystoscopy from computed tomography: a pilot study. *BJU Int* 2004; **94**(6): 828–31.

24. Kim J K, Ahn J H, Park T *et al*. Virtual cystoscopy of the contrast material-filled bladder in patients with gross hematuria. *AJR Am J Roentgenol* 2002; **179**(3): 763–8.

25. Kim J K, Park S Y, Kim H S *et al*. Comparison of virtual cystoscopy, multiplanar reformation, and source CT images with contrast material-filled bladder for detecting lesions. *AJR Am J Roentgenol* 2005; **185**(3): 689–96.

26. Schreyer A G, Fielding J R, Warfield S K *et al*. Virtual CT cystoscopy: color mapping of bladder wall thickness. *Invest Radiol* 2000; **35**(5): 331–4.

27. Fielding J R, Hoyte L X, Okon S A *et al*. Tumor detection by virtual cystoscopy with color mapping of bladder wall thickness. *J Urol* 2002; **167**(2 Pt 1): 559–62.

28. Beer A, Saar B, Rummeny E J. Tumors of the urinary bladder: technique, current use, and perspectives of MR and CT cystography. *Abdom Imaging* 2003; **28**(6): 868–76.

29. Lammle M, Beer A, Settles M *et al*. Reliability of MR imaging-based virtual cystoscopy in the diagnosis of cancer of the urinary bladder. *AJR Am J Roentgenol* 2002; **178**(6): 1483–8.

30. Wong-You-Cheong J J, Woodward P J, Manning M A *et al*. From the archives of the AFIP: neoplasms of the urinary bladder: radiologic-pathologic correlation. *Radiographics* 2006; **26**(2): 553–80.

31. Montironi R, Lopez-Beltran A. The 2004 WHO classification of bladder tumors: a summary and commentary. *Int J Surg Pathol* 2005; **13**(2): 143–53.

32. Shokeir A A. Squamous cell carcinoma of the bladder: pathology, diagnosis and treatment. *BJU Int* 2004; **93**(2): 216–20.

33. Thali-Schwab C M, Woodward P J, Wagner B J. Computed tomographic appearance of urachal adenocarcinomas: review of 25 cases. *Eur Radiol* 2005; **15**(1): 79–84.

34. Hughes M J, Fisher C, Sohaib S A. Imaging features of primary nonurachal adenocarcinoma of the bladder. *AJR Am J Roentgenol* 2004; **183**(5): 1397–401.

35. Bates A W, Norton A J, Baithun S I. Malignant lymphoma of the urinary bladder: a clinicopathological study of 11 cases. *J Clin Pathol* 2000; **53**(6): 458–61.

36. Sahdev A, Sohaib A, Monson J P *et al*. CT and MR imaging of unusual locations of extra-adrenal paragangliomas (pheochromocytomas). *Eur Radiol* 2005; **15**(1): 85–92.

37. Umaria N, Olliff J F. MRI appearances of bladder endometriosis. *Br J Radiol* 2000 July; **73**(871): 733–6. PMID: 11089464.

4

Radiological staging of primary bladder cancer

Camilla Whitten and David MacVicar

Introduction

Bladder cancer is a common tumor of the urinary tract. Staging of disease is important as it gives some indication of prognosis and helps determine clinical management. It also allows some comparison of treatment response and comparison between patients [1].

Staging of bladder cancer is based on depth of tumor invasion of the bladder wall, involvement of local structures, nodal involvement and metastases. The bladder can be divided into layers: The mucosa (epithelium) lies over the submucosa or lamina propria. Beneath this is the muscular layer and beyond this is the serosa (the serosa is not present over the entire bladder as it is synonymous with the peritoneal covering which is applied over the dome) [2–4]. Staging systems for local disease are based on these layers. There are two main staging classifications used for evaluating bladder carcinoma: the TNM classification [5] and the Jewett–Strong–Marshall classification [6]. The TNM classification was revised in 1997, with a new stage added to differentiate between microscopic and macroscopic perivesical disease, a modification which has been retained in more recent versions (Table 4.1).

Clinical staging is evaluated by a combination of imaging, bimanual palpation, cystoscopic evaluation and biopsy [1,2]. Ideally, imaging would be performed prior to cystoscopy and biopsy to minimize potential imaging artifacts. In practice, however, cystoscopy and biopsy are performed at the initial presentation. Cystoscopic resection may completely remove the tumor and allow staging based on the histology (see Chapter 1). In patients with more invasive disease, imaging may provide additional information to that obtained by bimanual assessment [2].

Carcinoma of the Bladder, ed. David MacVicar. Published by Cambridge University Press. © Cambridge University Press 2008.

Table 4.1. TNM Classification for bladder cancer [5]

TX	Primary tumor cannot be assessed
T0	No evidence of primary tumor
Ta	Non-invasive papillary carcinoma
Tis	Carcinoma *in situ*: "flat tumor"
T1	Tumor invades subepithelial connective tissue
T2	Tumor invades muscle
T2a	Tumor invades superficial muscle (inner half)
T2b	Tumor invades deep muscle (outer half)
T3	Tumor invades perivesical tissue
T3a	microscopically
T3b	macroscopically (extravesical mass)
T4	Tumor invades any of the following: prostate, uterus, vagina, pelvic wall, abdominal wall
T4a	Tumor invades prostate or uterus or vagina
T4b	Tumor invades pelvic wall or abdominal wall
NX	Regional lymph nodes cannot be assessed
N0	No regional lymph node metastasis
N1	Metastasis in a single lymph node ≤ 2 cm in greatest dimension
N2	Metastasis in a single lymph node >2 cm but ≤ 5 cm in greatest dimension, or multiple lymph nodes, none >5 cm in greatest dimension
N3	Metastasis in a lymph node >5 cm in greatest dimension
MX	Distant metastases cannot be assessed
M0	No distant metastases
M1	Distant metastases

Local staging of bladder cancer

Computed tomography

Certain criteria have been used in studies to attempt staging of bladder cancer on CT: a superficial tumor may be seen as a pedunculated lesion (T1 or less), sessile lesions have been designated superficial muscle invasive (T2a) and a sessile lesion with wall thickening suggests deep muscle invasion (T2b) [7–9]. However, despite these attempts, CT has proved unsatisfactory for evaluating depth of involvement of organ-confined disease and its main role is to distinguish organ-confined tumors from those spreading into the perivesical fat (T3). Perivesical fat infiltration is seen as an irregular, shaggy border of the bladder with streaky areas of

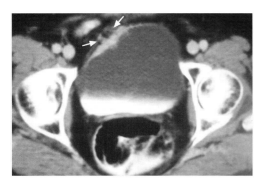

Figure 4.1 CT scan following intravenous contrast. Some delay has occurred, resulting in pooling of contrast in the posterior bladder. There is a diffuse mass thickening the anterior bladder wall to the right of the midline. Irregular enhancing tissue is seen extending into the perivesical fat (arrows), giving a "shaggy" outline indicative of extravesical spread, stage T3b.

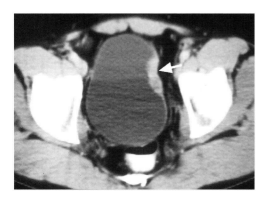

Figure 4.2 CT scan of bladder following intravenous contrast. There is an enhancing mass on the left lateral bladder wall. There is some apparent retraction of the outline of the urinary bladder (arrow). An appearance such as this is difficult to interpret as the perivesical fat is essentially normal and there is no convincing evidence of an extravesical mass lesion. Subsequently cystectomy demonstrated extravesical spread, disease stage T3b (reproduced with permission of Taylor & Francis (Informa plc) from *Imaging in Oncology*, 2nd edn, Husband J E, Reznek R H (eds.), 2004, 17.4).

higher attenuation in the fat (Fig. 4.1), or a perivesical mass [7–10]. Most studies in the literature were performed prior to the 1997 change in the TNM staging system and did not address the difficult problem of assessing for microscopic or macroscopic disease, which are now assigned different stages (T3a versus T3b in the TNM system) (Fig. 4.2). Invasion of adjacent organs (T4a) is often difficult to confirm by imaging as the tumor may be in contact with the organ but not invading it; however, if the tumor mass is directly extending into the adjacent structure, invasion is implied [2,11] (Fig. 4.3). Assessment of some of the surrounding fat planes may also help. There is usually an angle between the seminal vesicle and the bladder, which is filled with fat. If tumor invades the seminal vesicle, the fat will be obscured [2,12]. Some false positive investigations may result from an over-distended bladder or rectum causing filling in of the fat plane, mimicking seminal vesicle invasion (note that the TNM system does not specify the seminal vesicles as an adjacent organ) (Fig. 4.4) [12]. Invasion of the pelvic sidewall or abdominal wall

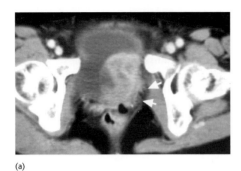
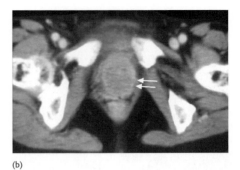

(a)   (b)

Figure 4.3 (a) CT scan of bladder with intravenous contrast. There is an enhancing mass postero-laterally on the left which demonstrates an intraluminal component and full thickness involvement of the bladder wall with an irregular outline of the mass extending toward the pelvic sidewall (arrows). Proximity to the obturator muscle raises the possibility of pelvic sidewall invasion (reproduced with permission of Husband J E, Reznek R H, from *Imaging in Oncology*, 1st edn, 1998, 14.8(a). (b) Images caudally to Figure 4.3a demonstrate that the mass has extended peri-urethrally into the pelvic floor, where there is evidence of involvement of the pelvic floor muscles (arrows). Disease stage T4b.

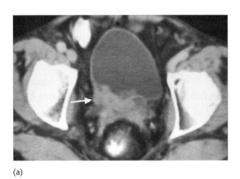
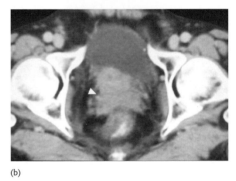

(a)   (b)

Figure 4.4 CT scan of pelvis with intravenous contrast. (a) A mass lesion is present on the posterior wall of the urinary bladder. There is evidence of an extravesical mass (arrow). (b) The angle between the bladder and the seminal vesicles has been obliterated and there is invasion of the seminal vesicles (arrowhead). Within the TNM system, involvement of adjacent organs is designated T4a, although gut and seminal vesicles are not specifically identified as adjacent organs.

constitutes stage T4b disease and some studies considered this was present if the perivesical spread was seen to extend to within 3 mm of the pelvic sidewall or was inseparable from the pelvic sidewall muscles (Figs. 4.3 and 4.5) [10]. However, there are limitations of CT with an overall accuracy of 35–55% for staging bladder cancer (with one study reporting sensitivity of 95% and specificity of 28% [13]) and it is not possible to distinguish between stages of superficial bladder cancer (Ta and T1) [7–9,13–15]. Differentiating organ-confined disease from non–organ-confined

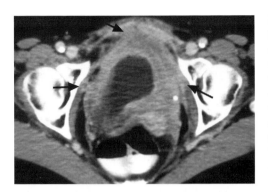

Figure 4.5 CT scan of bladder following intravenous contrast. There is gross thickening of most of the wall of the urinary bladder. Mucosal irregularity is present, enhancing tumor replaces the full thickness of the wall, and there is enhancing tissue extending into the pelvic sidewalls bilaterally and also the anterior abdominal wall (arrows). Disease stage T4b (reproduced with permission of Husband J E, Reznek R H, from *Imaging in Oncology*, 1st edn, 1998, 14.17(a)).

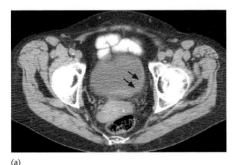

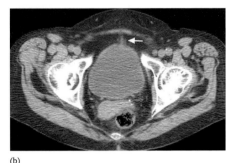

(a)   (b)

Figure 4.6 CT scan with intravenous contrast, following transurethral resection of bladder tumor with multiple biopsies. (a) demonstrates diffuse thickening of the posterior and left lateral bladder wall (arrows). Histology indicated invasion of the muscularis propria (pT2a, at least) by grade 3 transitional cell carcinoma. (b) Slightly caudal to the previous image, demonstrates streaking of the perivesical fat anteriorly at the site of biopsy performed by cystoscopic procedure (arrow). An appearance such as this is not confirmatory of extravesical spread, but clinical correlation is necessary to establish that this may be a treatment-related appearance. Comorbidity and patient preference led to treatment with radical radiotherapy, and the patient remains disease-free at two years for presumed T2 organ-confined disease.

disease has an accuracy of 64–87% on CT [7,9,10,16–18] and in some studies sensitivities of 60–94% and specificities of 62–100% have been reported [9,10,18]. The majority of discrepancies in histologically correlated series appear to be due to overstaging [7,9,10,13,14].

Demonstration of early extravesical spread and early organ invasion may be problematical [10,11,19]. It is frequently not possible to differentiate edema or treatment-induced changes from extravesical tumor extension (Fig. 4.6) [10]. Tumor location may also affect CT evaluation as tumors at the dome and trigone have historically been difficult to assess with axial scanning (though this difficulty may be reduced by the availability of multislice CT with multiplanar reformatting) (Fig. 4.7).

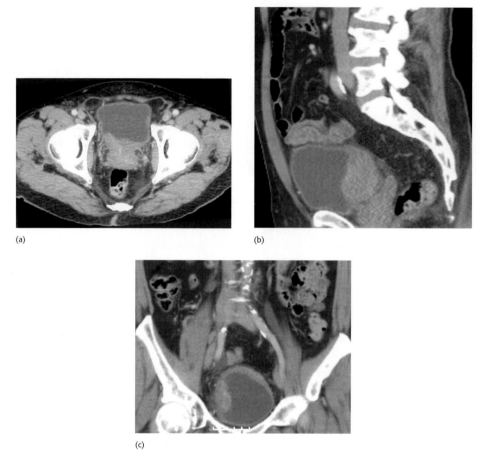

(a)

(b)

(c)

Figure 4.7 (a) Axial CT following intravenous contrast, through inferior bladder. There is thickening of the posterior wall of the bladder close to the prostate. (b) Sagittal reformat demonstrates bulky tumor with extensive thickening of the posterior bladder wall. However, there is no definite evidence of prostatic invasion and a fat plane is identifiable between bladder tumor and seminal vesicles. Likewise there is no confirmatory evidence of involvement of the small bowel lying superior to the bladder. (c) Coronal oblique reformat demonstrating tumor on the posterior wall of the bladder is almost circumferential. The irregular outline signifies that some degree of perivesical fat infiltration is present, indicating T3 disease. Cystoprostatectomy confirmed pT3b disease, but without invasion of prostate or seminal vesicles.

Bladder tumors can be assessed with contrast-enhanced CT scans, and enhancement of the intraluminal and extraluminal component can facilitate delineation of the extent of disease [10]. Newer bladder imaging techniques such as CT cystography and virtual cystoscopy have been employed to detect bladder abnormalities [20–24]. These techniques can also provide information on the extent of extravesical disease [21–23]. Wang *et al.* [24] have formally assessed staging using axial and multiplanar reconstruction (MPR) images derived from helical CT with 3D reconstructions and virtual cystoscopy. Using MPR and axial images, there was a reported overall staging accuracy of 87.7% though it is not clear whether subdivisions of superficial and deep muscle invasion were applied in the calculation. An accuracy of 94.7% was achieved for staging non–organ-confined disease. Extravesical extension and its relationship to the ureters could be assessed on the MPR images. The 3D reconstructions could partially reveal extravesical information but not as clearly as the axial and MPR images, and virtual cystoscopy images did not provide information on the extravesical tumor component [24].

Some authors have evaluated bladder wall infiltration with the bladder filled with different contrast media such as unopacified urine, urine opacified with iodinated contrast and air-insufflation [25]. The authors of this study found the air-insufflation technique the most accurate for staging, with an overall accuracy of 95%, and the unopacified urine technique the least accurate, with an overall accuracy of 87%. The majority of inaccuracies, as in other CT studies, were due to overstaging. Organ-confined, muscle invasive disease was the least accurately staged disease. The study used spiral CT and the authors noted their reported accuracies were higher than those previously cited in the literature, which they attributed to technological advances since previous studies and their efforts to distend the bladder. However, the bladder insufflation technique is invasive, requiring the patient to be catheterized. In addition, the authors of the study acknowledged that tumors had a tendency to be overstaged when the bladder contained unopacified or opacified urine in comparison to air insufflation due to difficulty in achieving optimal bladder distension [25]. This raises the question whether the apparent improvement in staging accuracy was due to the negative contrast medium of air or due to the degree of bladder distension. An earlier study using carbon dioxide to distend the bladder resulted in an accuracy of 81% in distinguishing organ-confined from non–organ-confined disease [26]. Olive oil has also been used to fill the bladder in CT assessment of bladder tumors [9].

Magnetic resonance imaging

On T1-weighted imaging, bladder tumors are seen as intermediate signal intensity masses, returning signal with intensity similar to that of the bladder wall [4,10,18,27]. The mucosa and muscle are not differentiated [15]. As a result, problems arise in attempting to stage disease confined to the bladder wall on

T1-weighted imaging. However, tumor spread beyond the bladder wall is seen on T1-weighted imaging and is demonstrable as soft tissue contiguous with the primary tumor and of similar signal intensity (Fig. 4.8) [10]. The tumor may have a wispy appearance or be a solid mass, but will normally contrast with the signal returned from surrounding fat [16,28].

On T2-weighted imaging, the normal bladder wall is identified as a hypointense line outlining the bladder lumen [8,29–31]. This is thought to represent the muscle layer [32]. Some authors report an inner band of low signal intensity and an outer band of intermediate signal intensity in the bladder wall on T2-weighted imaging and attribute this to a compact inner and looser outer layer arrangement of smooth muscle fibers (Fig. 4.9) [32]. Bladder tumors return signal of intensity higher than that of the adjacent normal bladder wall [4,10,11,15,18,27]. The tumor can therefore be distinguished from the bladder muscle [15,31,33] and an attempt at assessing depth of muscle infiltration can be made (Figs. 4.10–4.12). Involvement of the seminal vesicles can be assessed on T2-weighted images, with low signal intensity tumor replacing the normal high signal intensity fluid in the seminal vesicles [10,16]. Evidence of fat invasion in the angle between the seminal vesicle and bladder wall may also be seen [16]. Invasion of other adjacent organs such as the prostate and cervix is best assessed on the T2-weighted sequence [11].

On dynamic contrast-enhanced MRI, bladder tumors show moderate enhancement and are higher in signal intensity than the background bladder [7]. Tumor, mucosa and submucosa enhance on the images taken immediately after intravenous (IV) gadolinium whereas the muscle layer remains hypointense [8,15,27,29]. Narumi *et al.* [34] showed the maximum contrast–noise ratio between tumor and bladder wall was achieved in the earliest imaging phase (0–95 seconds). On delayed images there is less contrast between the muscle layer and tumor [7, 27,34]. Dynamic

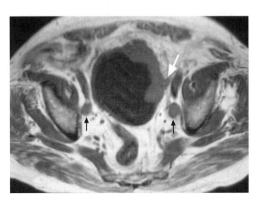

Figure 4.8 T1-weighted axial MRI of bladder. There is a mass replacing the bladder wall to the left of the midline. There is extension into the perivesical fat (white arrow). Note also bilateral obturator nodes which return similar signal to the bladder tumor and perivesical extension (black arrows).

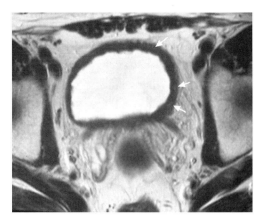

Figure 4.9 T2-weighted axial MRI through urinary bladder in a patient with benign prostatic hypertrophy causing thickening of the bladder wall. There is no history of bladder carcinoma. The image demonstrates hypertrophied low signal muscle layer. Peripherally, there is some slightly increased signal (arrows), which some authors have attributed to the muscle fibres in the outer detrusor being more loosely packed compared with the inner detrusor. This inhomogeneity of signal is observed, but is not reliably reproducible, and in the authors' opinion is unreliable in trying to discriminate between superficial and deep muscle invasion by tumor (reproduced with permission of Taylor & Francis (Informa plc) from *Imaging in Oncology*, 2nd edn, Husband J E, Reznek R H (eds.), 2004, 17.14(d)).

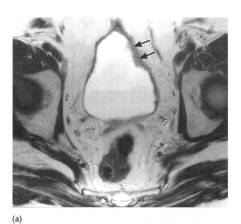

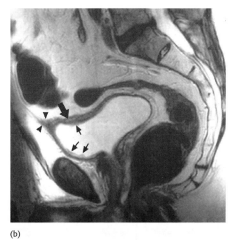

(a)   (b)

Figure 4.10 T2-weighted MRI in axial and sagittal plane. Cystoscopy had revealed multifocal superficial tumor. (a) Axial image demonstrates disease along the left lateral wall of the bladder. Low signal from the muscularis is evident posteriorly, but anteriorly and to the left of the midline there is clear evidence of mucosal tumor, which appears to be penetrating into the muscularis (arrows). (b) Sagittal image demonstrates low signal of the muscularis posteriorly, but more anteriorly there is extensive intermediate signal along the mucosa (small arrows) which infiltrates through the wall (large arrow), and also into the perivesical fat (arrowheads). Although in most places disease is superficial or confined to the muscularis, by imaging criteria disease stage would be T3b (reproduced with permission of Taylor & Francis (Informa plc) from *Imaging in Oncology*, 2nd edn, Husband J E, Reznek R H (eds.), 2004, 17.17(c)).

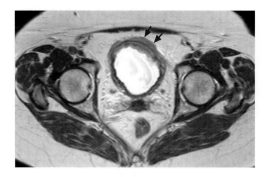

Figure 4.11 Axial T2-weighted MRI of bladder at the level of the acetabulum. There is extensive tumor. Postero-laterally to the left there is low signal from the muscularis. A mass lying laterally to the left of the midline extending anteriorly demonstrates an intraluminal component and also extravesical spread. Low signal from the muscle continues through the mass, but there is clear evidence of abnormal signal within the muscle layer, indicating infiltration through the wall into the perivesical fat (arrows).

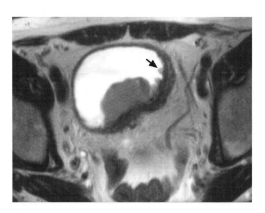

Figure 4.12 Axial T2-weighted MRI of bladder. A large polypoid tumor is present on the posterior wall of the bladder. Further small polypoid tumors are present on the left lateral bladder wall (arrow). Tumor signal does not extend into the muscularis, which is noted to be thickened. This thickening is non-specific, and does not confirm extravesical spread. Disease is therefore considered to be organ confined. Following chemotherapy and radiotherapy, complete remission was obtained and the patient remains disease-free at six years.

MRI may therefore have some potential in discriminating muscle from tumor and thus staging disease confined to the wall. One downside to dynamic imaging in some reported studies has been the limited field of view and the restriction to one imaging plane obtained for assessment [35], but the available technology continues to evolve. It is noted that in some non-dynamic MRI studies, enhanced images did not always provide more information than the conventional sequences [36].

Using a combination of a STIR (Short Tau Inversion Recovery, a pulse sequence that suppresses the signal from fat) sequence with air insufflation of the bladder, the bladder wall can be delineated between a nulled signal from the perivesical fat and a signal void from the lumen [35]. Tumor can be identified by the return of signal of intensity different from that of the bladder wall signal and attempts have been made to stage bladder cancer using this technique. The authors of the study demonstrated non-muscle invasive disease, with histopathologic correlation, and with an identification accuracy of 79.2%. They also correctly identified full thickness invasion of the muscle in a very high proportion of patients. However, they did not attempt to separate perivesical extension from deep muscle invasion in this group and therefore the clinical utility of the technique and reported accuracy are relatively limited [35].

Certain imaging criteria applied to T2-weighted and contrast-enhanced MRI have emerged from the literature. An intact, linear, low signal intensity muscle layer at the base of the tumor leads to classification as T1 or less; an irregular inner margin of the low signal intensity muscle layer as T2a; and a disrupted low signal intensity muscle layer without perivesical infiltration is classified as T2b [7–9, 29,34]. A lesion with an irregular, shaggy outer border and streaky areas of the same signal intensity as the primary tumor in the perivesical fat, or a perivesical mass, is staged as T3b (Figs. 4.13–4.15) [18,29,34,37]; however, T1-weighting (unenhanced) is often better at demonstrating extravesical extension [8,10,18,36]. Tumor within a diverticulum is categorized as T3, as there is no muscle layer (Fig. 4.16). Extension of an imaging-detectable mass with abnormal signal into an adjacent organ [10,18] is considered T4a and that into the abdominal or pelvic sidewalls is considered T4b (Figs. 4.17–4.19) [29,37]. A number of studies were performed prior to 1997, when revision of TNM staging introduced stage T3a as indicative of microscopically detected extravesical spread, and there is limited literature since that time.

When reviewing the literature for statistics regarding MRI in bladder cancer staging, a number of factors should be borne in mind. The size of studies and

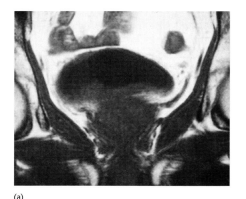
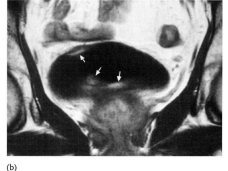

(a)   (b)

Figure 4.13 T1-weighted coronal MRI (a) before and (b) after gadolinium enhancement. Pre-contrast images show some thickening of the wall of the bladder superiorly and around the trigone. Following contrast, there are areas of focal enhancement superficially (arrows). There is no evidence of an extravesical mass, and this appearance represents superficial organ-confined disease.

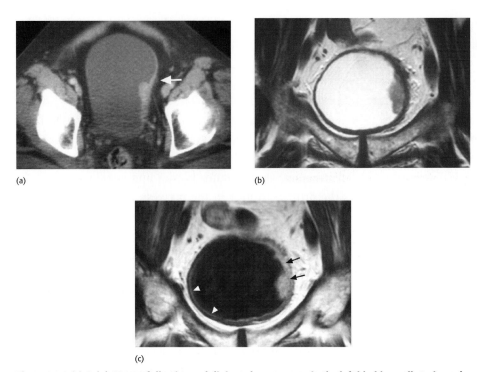

(a)   (b)

(c)

Figure 4.14 **(a) Axial CT scan following gadolinium shows a mass in the left bladder wall. An irregular outline is noted, suspicious of perivesical fat infiltration (arrow). (b) T2-weighted coronal MRI confirms the mass on the left bladder wall. Abnormal signal extends into the muscle layer, but the appearance is equivocal for extravesical spread (reproduced with permission of Taylor & Francis (Informa plc) from** *Imaging in Oncology,* **2nd edn, Husband J E, Reznek R H (eds.), 2004, 17.16(a)). (c) Gadolinium-enhanced T1-weighted coronal image demonstrates enhancement penetrating the muscle layer. Abnormal enhancement of the wall (arrows) suggests that disease is more widespread than evident on T2-weighted imaging. Edema and post-treatment change can result in abnormal signal or enhancement characteristics within the bladder wall, but the extent of the enhancement and the presence of an irregular outline to the lateral bladder wall led to staging as T3b tumor. Note also the normal linear enhancement of the mucosa and submucosa elsewhere in the bladder (arrowheads) on these early post-contrast images (reproduced with permission of Taylor & Francis (Informa plc) from** *Imaging in Oncology,* **2nd edn, Husband J E, Reznek R H (eds.), 2004, 17.16(c)).**

case-mix of disease stage within them is highly variable. The authors in the majority of studies report accuracy rather than the sensitivity and specificity. Modern technological advances have been made throughout the time course of articles appearing in the literature and therefore there is no standardized equipment, e.g. varying field strengths have been used and new coils such as the double surface coil and endorectal coils have been introduced, as opposed to the body coil imaging which was used in earlier studies. In addition, the bladder is an ever-changing

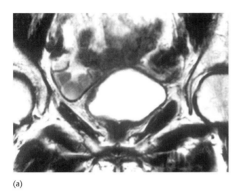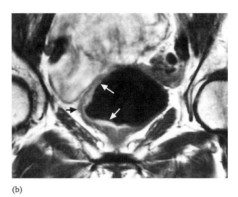

(a)   (b)

Figure 4.15 (a) T2-weighted coronal and (b) T1-weighted post-gadolinium coronal MRI. T2-weighted images show abnormal signal of the mucosa with probable extension into the muscularis on the right lateral bladder wall extending down to the bladder base. Following contrast, there is extensive enhancement at the bladder base and throughout the full thickness of the bladder wall (white arrows). There is some irregular tissue evident in the perivesical fat (black arrow), indicating a high likelihood of extravesical spread. Signal from the muscularis to the left of the midline is normal (Fig. 4.15a is reproduced with permission of Husband J E, Reznek R H, from *Imaging in Oncology*, 1st edn, 1998, 14.13(b)).

structure with respect to its distension. Given the relatively long scanning times involved in MRI, a balance must be struck between the bladder being distended well enough to visualize anatomy and the bladder not being so full as to be uncomfortable. Various methods have been described in the literature to optimize bladder filling, including patients not being allowed to void for a varying amount of time prior to the scan (e.g. 45 minutes or two hours [14,15]) or instructing patients to drink a fixed volume in a fixed time after they have voided [34].

Overall accuracy rates of 58–85% for staging with conventional MRI have been reported [7–9,14,18,27,34,38–40]. Incorporating dynamic imaging into the MRI assessment has reported accuracy rates of 62–85% [7,8,15,27,29,34,38,41], whereas using delayed-enhanced images results in lower reported accuracies of 56–74% [7,8,27]. Barentsz *et al.* [41] also evaluated a T1-weighted 3D imaging technique using a 3D MP-RAGE sequence, in addition to conventional and dynamic contrast-enhanced sequences, and the overall accuracy of staging improved from 78% to 93% with this additional sequence. Various authors have noted the difficulty in differentiating between superficial and deep muscle invasion [7,36] and have often concentrated on distinguishing if muscle invasion is present or not. Differentiating muscle invasive disease from non-muscle invasive disease with dynamic MRI has a reported accuracy of 85–92% [27,29,34] with one study reporting a sensitivity of 96.2% and specificity of 83.3% [15]. Assessing if tumors are organ confined or not

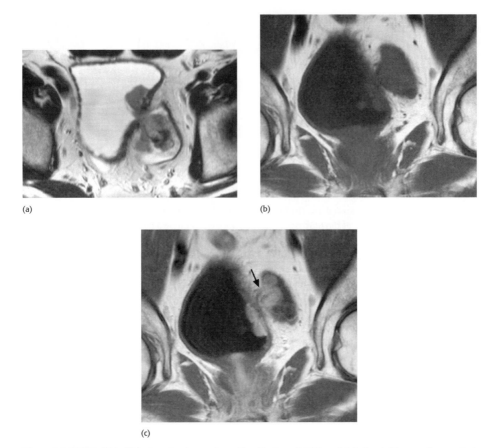

(a)   (b)

(c)

Figure 4.16 MRI of bladder showing tumor in a diverticulum. (a) T2-weighted axial image demonstrates polypoid tumor extending into bladder lumen. Tumor is also seen to enter a bladder diverticulum, and the full extent of tumor will be concealed from the cystoscope. Tumor within a diverticulum is staged T3 under most circumstances as the muscle layer is absent from the diverticulum. (b) and (c) Pre- and post-gadolinium T1-weighted coronal images. On the post-contrast image, enhancing tumor is demonstrated along the left lateral bladder wall entering the diverticulum (arrow). Streaking of perivesical fat is also in evidence consistent with extravesical spread of disease.

has a range of reported accuracy of 73–85% [7,9,10,16,18] on conventional MRI (with some studies reporting sensitivities of 60–83% and specificities of 62–100% [7,9,10,18]). For dynamic contrast-enhanced MRI, accuracies of 81–82% are reported [7,29] and with delayed-enhanced imaging, accuracies of 70–86% have been achieved [7,28]. CT and MRI have comparable accuracies for detecting perivesical extension [7,9]. MRI is said to be better than CT at evaluating seminal vesicle involvement [14,16]. The development of surface coils has improved the accuracy of staging bladder cancer in comparison to using the body coil only [40]. The

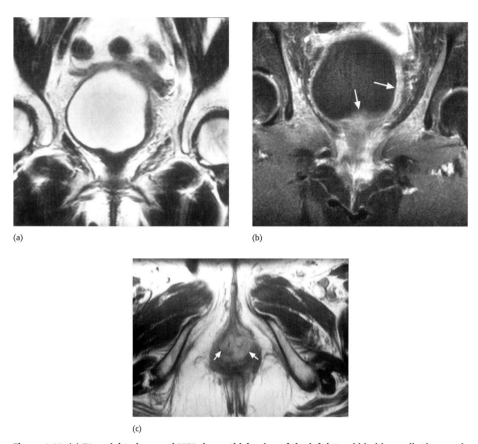

(a)

(b)

(c)

Figure 4.17 (a) T2-weighted coronal MRI shows thickening of the left lateral bladder wall. Abnormal signal is present throughout the bladder wall, suspicious of extravesical spread. (b) Fat-suppressed gadolinium-enhanced T1-weighted coronal MRI of bladder shows extensive abnormal signal in the bladder wall to the left of the midline extending to the bladder base and peri-urethrally (arrows) (reproduced with permission of Husband J E, Reznek R H, from *Imaging in Oncology*, 1st edn, 1998 14.19(b)). (c) In view of the suspicion of peri-urethral spread, further T1-weighted axial MR images were obtained following gadolinium, which demonstrate a mass lesion surrounding the urethra close to perineal level (arrows), indicating disease stage T4a (reproduced with permission of Husband J E, Reznek R H (eds.), from *Imaging in Oncology*, 1st edn, 1998, 14.19(d)).

multiplanar capability of MRI allows the extent of tumors in certain locations to be better visualized than on CT, in particular the bladder base and dome [7,8,14,42]. The majority of errors are attributed to overstaging [7,10,15,27,29,34,35], although this is not the case in all studies [18].

There are a number of pitfalls in interpreting MRI staging of bladder cancer. Despite technical advances, MRI cannot assess histology and difficulty remains in distinguishing tumor infiltration from inflammatory and post-biopsy changes in

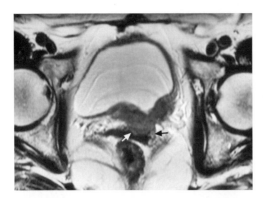

Figure 4.18 T2-weighted axial MRI of bladder demonstrating a tumor of the bladder wall lying posteriorly and to the left of the midline. There is unequivocal evidence of an extravesical mass. The tumor is also seen to be invading the upper vagina (arrows). Disease stage T4a by MRI criteria.

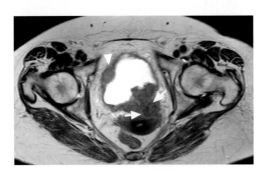

Figure 4.19 Multifocal bladder cancer. T2-weighted axial MRI shows a bulky mass with an intraluminal component, full thickness involvement of the bladder and an extravesical mass which is invading the uterus just above the level of the cervix (arrows). There is also a further mass anteriorly, to the right of the midline (arrowhead).

both the muscle and perivesical tissues [7,10,29,34,39]. Although improved image resolution may improve detection of perivesical fat stranding it still cannot reliably determine its cause [29]. Caution in attempting staging after recent biopsy is recommended [7]. It is also not possible to demonstrate microscopic invasion on MRI [34,37]. The thinness of the bladder wall makes accurate assessment regarding the depth of invasion difficult [7,9]. Judgment of the depth of muscle invasion is also affected by the degree of bladder distension [8,27]. If the bladder is overfilled, the wall is thinned, making detection of muscular disruption difficult [8,15,27,34]. If the bladder is collapsed, the mucosa and submucosa can show irregularity mimicking muscle invasion or distortion of the bladder wall and can give the impression of extension into perivesical tissues [8,27,43]. To obtain a constant and optimally distended bladder, controlled bladder filling with a urethral catheter during imaging would be ideal [34]. However, this is invasive and optimal patient preparation prior to the examination is a more practical approach, although the best protocol for achieving this is debatable. Partial volume effect at the tumor–bladder wall interface may lead to overstaging and can be avoided by optimizing the imaging plane by using an oblique plane through the tumor,

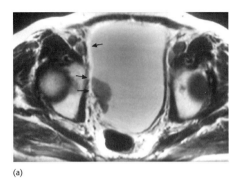
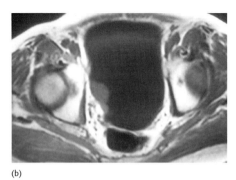

(a)   (b)

Figure 4.20 (a) T2-weighted axial MRI shows a mass lesion on the right bladder wall. Staging is compromised by a chemical shift artifact which has a generated a high signal line, obscuring the right bladder wall (arrows) (reproduced with permission of Husband J E, Reznek R H, from *Imaging in Oncology*, 1st edn, 1998, 14.11(c)), (b) T1-weighted axial MRI demonstrates the intra-luminal tumor mass, but no confirmatory evidence of extravesical spread. Changing phase encoding directions, using orthogonal planes and different sequences can overcome chemical shift artefact.

perpendicular to the bladder wall–tumor interface [34,43]. Chemical shift artifact, most often seen as a low signal intensity band along a lateral wall on one side and a high signal intensity band on the opposite side (Fig. 4.20), may obscure small tumors. The use of orthogonal plane imaging or changing the phase-encoding direction should overcome this potential pitfall [10,31,34]. If a low signal layer is generated by chemical shift artifact, care should be taken not to interpret it as a muscle layer [43]. When assessing contrast-enhanced images, inflow of urine from the ureteric orifices and inhomogeneous mixing of contrast and urine should not be mistaken for tumor, and comparison with other sequences and planes of imaging should be employed to eliminate this possible error [36].

Endorectal surface coils have also been assessed and an enhancing layer, pathologically confirmed as the submucosa, has been noted on scans performed five minutes post-contrast [44,45]. This submucosal linear enhancement (SLE) allows the bladder wall to be divided into three layers – the mucosa, submucosa and muscle [44,45]. Takeda *et al.* [45] acknowledge studies in the previous literature where post-contrast scans were performed immediately after contrast administration, demonstrating enhancement in both the mucosa and submucosa. However, they state the reason for detecting three layers in their study was that the mucosa could be seen as an unenhanced layer between the contrast-enhanced urine (seen within the bladder on their five-minute scans) and the submucosal enhancing layer, whereas previous studies had performed the scans early when the urine was not enhanced, which would make it impossible to distinguish between an unenhanced mucosal layer and unenhanced urine. If the SLE maintains continuity beneath the tumor, it is considered superficial disease and if the SLE is interrupted, the tumor is considered invasive [44,45]. A limitation to endorectal surface coils is tumor location. Tumors at the bladder neck, posterior, posterolateral and postero-inferior aspects of the bladder are well delineated. However, for assessment of anterior and superior bladder tumors, a combination with a pelvic phased-array coil is used. Hayashi *et al.* [44] found 83% of bladder tumors were correctly staged using the SLE and the accuracy of muscle invasion detection was 87%, with a sensitivity of 91% and specificity of 87%. The accuracy and specificity for detecting muscle invasion was significantly better than when using transurethral ultrasound [44]. Overstaging was once again noted to be the main source of error.

Maeda *et al.* [43] developed a technique which achieved submillimeter pixels, and in some patients three different signal intensity layers of the bladder wall may be discerned on T2-weighted imaging. Between two low signal intensity muscle layers is a middle layer which returns high signal intensity, interpreted as loose connective tissue between the muscle layers [43]. However, this appearance is not seen uniformly throughout the bladder wall and is not seen in all patients. As inflammatory cells and edema return high signal intensity and cannot be distinguished from tumor, the authors of this study used the presence of disruption of the outer muscle layer as evidence of muscle invasion, whereas the presence of inner muscle layer disruption only did not confidently predict muscle invasion. Using this criterion, they demonstrated an accuracy of 96.2%, sensitivity of 100% and specificity of 91.7% for the presence of muscle invasion [43]. In an earlier study, a "double black line" with an intervening higher signal intensity on T2-weighted imaging was reported in the bladder wall at the site of tumor in 7 of 30 patients [10]. Chemical shift artifact was not thought responsible. In two of these patients, there was no disruption of either the inner or outer black line and the tumor was limited to the superficial muscle in these patients. No pathologic correlation of this appearance was performed in the study and the authors could only postulate, and it is not certain if this appearance is due to the loose connective tissue between muscle layers [10]. Other authors have also observed a band of intermediate signal intensity between two bands of low signal intensity in the bladder wall on T2-weighted imaging [32], and in particular they noted that this appearance may be seen in patients with hypertrophic bladder walls, post-irradiation bladders and when the bladder is not fully distended.

An attempt to differentiate between true tumor involvement and adjacent inflammatory and post-biopsy change has been made by noting the enhancement times of tumor and benign changes. Barentsz *et al.* [38] considered a lesion to be malignant if enhancement commenced within 10 seconds of arterial vessel enhancement and considered it benign if its enhancement began later than 10 seconds. They found a significant difference in enhancement times, with the mean enhancement time of 6.5 seconds for tumors and 13.6 seconds for post-biopsy tissue. The more rapid enhancement of tumor compared to benign entities was attributed to neovascularization. The accuracy of differentiating tumor from post-biopsy effects increased from 79 to 90% and the specificity increased from 33 to 92% by using these criteria. A false positive interpretation was seen in granulation tissue with hyperemia. There are some structures which also show enhancement before the 10 seconds (including bowel, bone marrow, parametrium, uterus and benign prostatic hypertrophy). However, the bladder cancer enhances earlier than these structures and the normal structures can be identified on unenhanced images [38].

Ultrasound

Conventional transabdominal, transrectal and transvaginal ultrasound have been used to attempt staging of bladder cancer [13,46,47]; however, they have been largely superseded by CT and MRI [11]. Transrectal ultrasound has limitations, as tumors at the bladder dome, neck and beyond 10 cm of the probe are not imaged satisfactorily using this technique [46]. Transvaginal ultrasound allows tumors located on the anterior bladder wall and bladder neck to be scrutinized but those on the sidewalls are less amenable to detailed assessment [47]. The usefulness of other ultrasound techniques in the assessment of bladder cancer staging is not fully known, but there have been some studies involving small patient numbers.

An association has been seen between bladder tumor size and vascularity on color Doppler ultrasound assessment (with no vascularity seen in tumors smaller than 23–24 mm) [48,49]. However, there has not been any significant association demonstrated between the presence or pattern of Doppler findings of tumor vascularity and tumor stage or histological grade [48].

Using carbon dioxide microbubbles as ultrasound contrast, tumor visualization is reported to be improved in comparison to conventional ultrasonography [50]. The enhancement of bladder tumor is prolonged compared to normal tissue. The study was not specifically designed to assess staging accuracy for bladder cancer but noted some relevant findings. Lack of an apparent hyperechoic area in the adjacent bladder wall and base of the tumor on contrast ultrasound suggests absence of muscle invasion. Extravesical disease is well visualized [50]. However, differentiation between deep muscle invasion and extravesical spread can be difficult due to high echogenicity of the primary tumor after microbubble enhancement, which generates posterior scattered echoes which can obscure the deeper muscle in the region of interest.

Transurethral ultrasonography (TUUS) uses an ultrasound probe which can be inserted via a cystoscope sheath [51]. Various frequency probes have been used (5.5–10 MHz) [9,15,44,51–56]. This technique also allows evaluation of bladder diverticula when the cystoscope cannot be passed into the diverticulum [51,52]. The whole thickness of the bladder wall has a uniform echogenicity and no distinction between the muscle layer and the mucosa or submucosa can be seen [51–53]. Tumors are seen as masses of mixed echogenicity that are less echogenic than the mucosa and muscle [53]. If there is no interruption of the normal, uniform echogenicity of the underlying bladder wall, a superficial tumor is suggested [9,51,53,54]. Muscle invasion is suggested when there is disruption of the uniform echogenicity of the bladder wall, and when this is organ confined, the thickness of the bladder wall behind the tumor appears reduced [51,52]. In one study, all patients with invasive tumors had limited distensibility of the bladder wall at the site of tumor, assessed by different degrees of bladder filling [52]. With tumor extension into the perivesical fat, the whole thickness of the bladder wall is disrupted [51,52]. Allowing for the inability to differentiate between Ta and T1 disease, overall staging accuracies of 54.4–92.6% have been reported [9,15,44,51,52,55,56]. Koraitim *et al.* [52] found TUUS very accurate for staging superficial and organ-confined muscle invasive disease but a marked decrease in accuracy in staging non–organ-confined disease. Others have found transurethral ultrasound useful for differentiating muscle invasive from non–muscle invasive disease but have had difficulty assessing the depth of muscle involvement (because of the bladder wall width being obscured) [9,53,57]. T4 disease may not be adequately evaluated by TUUS owing to the lack of depth of penetration by high-frequency transducers and is better assessed by cross-sectional techniques [51]. Most staging errors in TUUS are attributed to overstaging [15,44,51,52,54–56]. Some potential pitfalls include shadowing from large papillary tumors being interpreted as invasion [51,55], and scarring from previous transurethral resection as tumor [51,54], although some authors have not found scar tissue to be problematic [55]. Shadowing from calcification on the tumor surface has also been reported [44,57]. The intramural ureters are seen as symmetrical defects or hypoechoic zones at the bladder base [51,53] and when assessing tumors in this region, care should be taken not to mistake them for muscular invasion [53]. Holm *et al.* [56]

also found it impossible to distinguish the sequelae of irradiation from residual tumor or recurrence.

Higher frequency ultrasound probes have also been assessed; however, the numbers involved are small. A 20 MHz miniature transducer passed through the working channel of the cystoscope allows the tumor to stay under direct vision [53,58] and this technique has been termed endoluminal ultrasonography (ELUS). Horiuchi *et al.* [58] could identify three layers of the normal bladder wall; the inner hyperechoic layer represented the mucosa and submucosa, the middle hypoechoic layer represented the muscle layer and the outer hyperechoic layer corresponded to the adventitia. However, in another study, Saga *et al.* [53] describe this differently; in some patients three layers could be depicted, with a hyperechogenic mucosa, hypoechogenic submucosa and hyperechogenic muscle layer being described; however, in most patients it was not possible to recognize the hypoechogenic submucosal layer. The reason for the apparent discrepancy in the findings between these studies is not clear. Despite this, in both studies it was still not possible to distinguish between stages Ta and T1 in the superficial tumors or between T2a and T2b in the muscle invasive tumors. The overall accuracy of distinguishing muscle invasive from non–muscle invasive tumor was 84.2–88% [53,58]. In one study, overstaging was the most common error, and in all of these cases the tumor was broad based and larger than 2 cm [58]. The low penetration of the ultrasound beam of high frequency transducers was thought to account for these inaccuracies and the authors of the study suggest that tumors larger than 2 cm are assessed by a different imaging method [58]. To the contrary, Saga *et al.* [53] did not find tumor size to affect staging accuracy. Instead they found tumor site may be more problematic as they could not accurately depict the tumor base in a tumor at the bladder neck and another tumor in a diverticulum. They attributed this to the difficulty in achieving perpendicular scanning planes at these sites despite the flexibility of the ELUS probe. Saga *et al.* also evaluated patients with both ELUS and TUUS and did not find any difference between the two with respect to staging between superficial and muscle invasive tumors. They postulated that ELUS may be superior to TUUS owing to the clinical benefits of ease of control of the probe under direct vision, thereby avoiding potential complications such as bladder or prostate injury [53]. More recently, a new ultrasonic cystofiberscope has been developed which has ultrasound and endoscopy functions combined in a single flexible probe [59]. The authors claim additional benefits of this system include bladder neck tumors being more easily assessed because of the flexibility of the scope. The authors noted that there are areas for possible technical improvement as the ultrasonic cystofiberscope has a narrow irrigation channel, which can impede assessment in those patients with active hematuria. In addition, there is only a single working channel and thus one cannot use biopsy forceps and irrigation simultaneously. As yet it is not known if there is any additional benefit in comparison with ELUS in bladder tumor staging [59].

The utility of transurethral ultrasound is likely to be in the distinction of non–muscle invasive from muscle invasive disease [51] although it is recognized that overstaging occurs. Computed tomography and MRI are superior in assessing non–organ-confined disease and lymph nodes, but the literature appears to indicate TUUS has the potential to provide more diagnostic information on the staging of organ-confined disease [52,57].

Wagner *et al.* [60] have described a further development in ultrasound which is that of 3D-rendering. A fully distended bladder is required (more than 300 ml). A suprapubic ultrasound is performed with a dedicated 3D transducer which mechanically sweeps the image plane through a pre-determined angle to acquire the data set. The computer software to produce a true virtual 3D reconstruction is used off-line. The authors claim that three layers of the wall can be visualized using this technique: the urothelium, the lamina propria and the muscle layer. For discrimination of T2 tumors from lower stage superficial tumors, a staging accuracy of 79% was reported. As with TUUS, overstaging was the main problem [60].

Isotope studies

Most of the studies in the literature relating to bladder cancer refer to ^{18}FDG-PET rather than PET-CT though they often correlate findings with cross-sectional imaging. Positron Emission Tomography (PET) is not valuable in morphological staging of primary bladder cancers as it is not possible to visualize the depth of invasion. The main drawback to ^{18}FDG-PET is urinary accumulation of FDG, which impacts on its usefulness in staging bladder cancer. However, PET appears to be more useful in assessment of lymph nodes and distant metastases.

A variety of techniques have been described utilizing other radiopharmaceuticals, none of which have entered mainstream practice at the time of writing. The amino acid methionine can be labelled with carbon-11 and, in the form of L-methyl-^{11}C-methionine, can be used as a tracer in PET examinations [61,62]. This is not primarily excreted in the urine. Ahlstrom *et al.* [61] found that ^{11}C-methionine was taken up by bladder tumors, but failed to detect primary lesions 1 cm or less. Uptake of ^{11}C-methionine in bowel mucosa caused difficulties in identification of metastatic disease in pelvic lymph nodes, and the authors suggested a hybrid technique also using [18]FDG-PET. Letocha et al. [62] found that in biopsy-proven tumor recurrence, ^{11}C-methionine PET did not detect any tumor, but it was noted that with bladder transitional cell carcinoma (TCC) on treatment with chemotherapy, ^{11}C-methionine PET was able to demonstrate a reduction in tumor size and metabolic activity.

[11]C can also be used to label choline. This radiopharmaceutical is said not to be excreted in urine [63], although in practice some urinary activity has been observed [64]. However, the high levels of activity which hamper the use of FDG-PET in the pelvis are absent, and it has been demonstrated that uptake of ^{11}C-choline in normal bladder wall is similar to the non-specific uptake seen in the intestine, rectum and prostate. ^{11}C-choline PET demonstrated bladder tumors, although a false positive was noted in a patient with an indwelling urinary catheter, and inflammatory changes were presumed to be responsible for this [64]. Lymph node metastases are detectable in the pelvis with this technique, the observed false negative studies being caused by micrometastases of 5 mm and less in lymph nodes. Pre-malignant lesions such as dysplasia and carcinoma *in situ* were not detected by ^{11}C-choline PET, but it was also observed that superficial cancers were undetectable [64]. The authors postulate that this may be due to the limited resolution of current scanners, or may be due to low uptake of choline by such superficial lesions. Gofrit et al. [65], using ^{11}C-choline PET-CT, have visualized carcinoma *in situ* and postulate that this is likely to be due to improved resolution and sensitivity of PET-CT compared to conventional PET. Picchio et al. [66] found that ^{11}C-choline PET performed better than CT in overall accuracy for lymph node assessment. The median size of PET positive nodes in this study was 14 mm, with the metastatic lesions within the lymph node measuring 5 mm and above. A disadvantage of any technique using ^{11}C labelling is the short physical half-life of the isotope (20 minutes) [66]. This means that an onsite cyclotron is necessary and at present this is unrealistic in most centers [64,66]. ^{18}F-labelled choline has been synthesized, but as with [18]FDG-PET, urinary activity is present [67].

Radioimmunoscintigraphy has been assessed in some studies involving a small number of patients. MUC1 mucin is a high molecular weight glycoprotein found on a variety of epithelial surfaces including bladder urothelium. MUC1 is abnormally glycosylated in some common malignancies, including bladder cancer, and cancer-associated MUC1 is structurally different to normal MUC1. C595 is a monoclonal antibody raised against the protein core of human epithelial MUC1. Studies have shown that MUC1 is abnormally expressed in the majority of invasive bladder tumors and metastatic lymph nodes, which stain strongly with C595 [68].

Radiopharmaceuticals (99m Technetium and 111-indium) can be attached to C595 [68,69]. It has been possible to visualize the primary mucosal tumor, lymph node metastases and distant metastases, including some lymph node metastases not detected on CT and MRI [69]. Simms *et al.* [68] reported a true positive rate of 80% using technetium-labelled C595. Drawbacks were observed with the technique when using both indium and technetium, including uptake in the liver and spleen and renal excretion. Some bladder activity is observed, and catheterization with bladder irrigation has been suggested as a remedy [68]. These results are interesting but the authors draw attention to the need for larger-scale prospective trials for further evaluation.

Conclusion

Staging by imaging investigations is a fundamental part of decision-making, particularly when radical treatment is being contemplated. Computed tomography and MRI remain the conventional techniques by which most staging is performed, and MRI retains certain advantages such as increased contrast resolution and direct multiplanar imaging. However, multidetector CT has produced an improvement in image quality and allows data manipulation to reconstruct multiple planes. It has the advantage of shorter examination times, particularly when whole body imaging is required. Other techniques including PET remain of unproven clinical utility.

REFERENCES

1. Gospodarowicz M K. Staging of bladder cancer. *Semin Surg Oncol* 1994; **10**: 51–9.
2. MacVicar A D. Bladder cancer staging. *BJU Int* 2000; **86**(suppl 1): 111–22.
3. Barentsz J O, Ruijs S H, Strijk S P. The role of MR imaging in carcinoma of the urinary bladder. *AJR Am J Roentgenol* 1993; **160**: 937–47.
4. Barentsz J O, Jager G J, Witjes J A, Ruijs J H. Primary staging of urinary bladder carcinoma: the role of MRI and a comparison with CT. *Eur Radiol* 1996; **6**: 129–33.
5. International Union Against Cancer. Sobin L H, Wittekind Ch, eds. *TNM Classification of Malignant Tumours* (6th edn). New York: Wiley-Liss, 2002.
6. Jewett H, Strong G. Infiltrating carcinoma of the bladder: relation of depth of penetration of the bladder wall to incidence of local extension in metastases. *J Urol* 1946; **55**: 366–72.
7. Kim B, Semelka R C, Ascher S M *et al*. Bladder tumour staging: comparison of contrast-enhanced CT, T1- and T2-weighted MR imaging, dynamic gadolinium-enhanced imaging, and late gadolinium-enhanced imaging. *Radiology* 1994; **193**: 239–45.

8. Tanimoto A, Yuasa Y, Imai Y *et al.* Bladder tumour staging: comparison of conventional and gadolinium-enhanced dynamic MR imaging and CT. *Radiology* 1992; **185**: 741–7.

9. Nishimura K, Hida S, Nishio Y *et al.* The validity of magnetic resonance imaging (MRI) in the staging of bladder cancer: comparison with computed tomography (CT) and transurethral ultrasonography (US). *Jpn J Clin Oncol* 1988; **18**: 217–26.

10. Husband J E, Olliff J F, Williams M P *et al.* Bladder cancer: staging with CT and MR imaging. *Radiology* 1989; **173**: 435–40.

11. Husband J E. Staging bladder cancer. *Clin Radiol* 1992; **46**: 153–9.

12. Freidland G W. Staging of genitourinary cancers. The role of diagnostic imaging. *Cancer* 1987; **60**: 450–8.

13. Yaman O, Baltaci S, Arikan N *et al.* Staging with computed tomography, transrectal ultrasonography and transurethral resection of bladder tumour: comparison with final pathological stage in invasive bladder carcinoma. *Br J Urol* 1996; **78**: 197–200.

14. Amendola M A, Glazer G M, Grossman H B *et al.* Staging of bladder carcinoma: MRI-CT-surgical correlation. *AJR Am J Roentgenol* 1986; **146**: 1179–83.

15. Tachibana M, Baba S, Deguchi N *et al.* Efficacy of gadolinium-diethylenetriaminepentaacetic acid-enhanced magnetic resonance imaging for differentiation between superficial and muscle-invasive tumour of the bladder: a comparative study with computerized tomography and transurethral Ultrasonography. *J Urol* 1991; **145**: 1169–73.

16. Bryan P J, Butler H E, LiPuma J P *et al.* CT and MR imaging in staging bladder neoplasms. *J Comput Assist Tomogr* 1987; **11**: 96–101.

17. Koss J C, Arger P H, Coleman B G *et al.* CT staging of bladder carcinoma. *AJR Am J Roentgenol* 1981; **137**: 359–62.

18. Buy J N, Moss A A, Guinet C *et al.* MR staging of bladder carcinoma: correlation with pathologic findings. *Radiology* 1988; **169**: 695–700.

19. Morgan C L, Calkins R F, Cavalcanti E J. Computed tomography in the evaluation, staging and therapy of carcinoma of the bladder and prostate. *Radiology* 1981; **140**: 751–61.

20. Browne R F, Murphy S M, Grainger R, Hamilton S. CT cystography and virtual cystoscopy in the assessment of new and recurrent bladder neoplasms. *Eur J Radiol* 2005; **53**: 147–53.

21. Yazgan C, Fitoz S, Atasoy C *et al.* Virtual cystoscopy in the evaluation of bladder tumours. *Clin Imaging* 2004; **28**: 138–42.

22. Tsili A Ch, Tsampoulas C, Chatziparaskevas N *et al.* Computed tomographic virtual cystoscopy for the detection of urinary bladder neoplasms. *Eur Radiol* 2004; **46**: 579–85.

23. Kawai N, Mimura T, Nagata D *et al.* Intravenous urography-virtual cystoscopy is a better preliminary examination than air virtual cystoscopy. *BJU Int* 2004; **94**: 832–6.

24. Wang D, Zhang W S, Xiong M H *et al.* Bladder tumours: dynamic contrast-enhanced axial imaging, multiplanar reformation, three-dimensional reconstruction and virtual cystoscopy using helical CT. *Chin Med J (Engl)* 2004; **117**: 62–6.

25. Caterino M, Giunta S, Finocchi V *et al*. Primary cancer of the urinary bladder: CT evaluation of the T parameter with different techniques. *Abdom Imaging* 2001; **26**: 433–8.

26. Seidelmann F E, Cohen W N, Bryan P J *et al*. Accuracy of CT staging of bladder neoplasms using the gas-filled method: report of 21 Patients with surgical confirmation. *AJR Am J Roentgenol* 1978; **130**: 735–9.

27. Scattoni V, Da Pozzo L F, Colombo R *et al*. Dynamic gadolinium-enhanced magnetic resonance imaging in staging of superficial bladder cancer. *J Urol* 1996; **155**: 1594–9.

28. Neuerburg J M, Bohndorf K, Sohn M *et al*. Staging of urinary bladder neoplasms with MR imaging: is Gd-DTPA helpful? *J Comput Assist Tomogr* 1991; **15**: 780–6.

29. Tekes A, Kamel I, Imam K *et al*. Dynamic MRI of bladder cancer: evaluation of staging accuracy. *AJR Am J Roentgenol* 2005; **184**: 121–7.

30. Fisher M R, Hricak H, Crooks L E. Urinary bladder MR imaging. Part I. Normal and benign conditions. *Radiology* 1985; **157**: 467–70.

31. Rholl K, Lee J K, Heiken J P *et al*. Primary bladder carcinoma: evaluation with MR imaging. *Radiology* 1987; **163**: 117–21.

32. Narumi Y, Kadota T, Inoue E *et al*. Bladder wall morphology: in vitro MR imaging-histopathologic correlation. *Radiology* 1993; **187**: 151–5.

33. Persad R, Kabala J, Gillatt D *et al*. Magnetic resonance imaging in the staging of bladder cancer. *Br J Urol* 1993; **71**: 566–73.

34. Narumi Y, Kadota T, Inoue E *et al*. Bladder tumors: staging with gadolinium-enhanced oblique MR imaging. *Radiology* 1993; **187**: 145–50.

35. Bartolozzi C, Caramella D, Zampa V *et al*. MR imaging with STIR technique and air insufflation for local staging of bladder neoplasms. *Acta Radiol* 1992; **33**: 577–81.

36. Hawnaur J M, Johnson R J, Read G, Isherwood I. Magnetic resonance imaging with gadolinium-DTPA for assessment of bladder carcinoma and its response to treatment. *Clin Radiol* 1993; **47**: 302–10.

37. Tavares N J, Demas B E, Hricak H. MR imaging of bladder neoplasms: correlation with pathologic staging. *Urol Radiol* 1990; **12**: 27–33.

38. Barentsz J O, Jager G J, van Vierzen P B *et al*. Staging urinary bladder cancer after transurethral biopsy: value of fast dynamic contrast-enhanced MR imaging. *Radiology* 1996; **201**: 185–93.

39. Fisher M R, Hricak H, Tanagho E A. Urinary bladder MR imaging: Part II. Neoplasm. *Radiology* 1985; **157**: 471–7.

40. Barentsz J O, Lemmens J A, Ruijs S H *et al*. Carcinoma of the urinary bladder: MR imaging with a double surface coil. *AJR Am J Roentgenol* 1988; **151**: 107–12.

41. Barentsz J O, Jager G, Mugler J P 3rd *et al*. Staging urinary bladder cancer: value of T1-weighted three-dimensional magnetization prepared-rapid gradient-echo and two-dimensional spin-echo sequences. *AJR Am J Roentgenol* 1995; **164**: 109–15.

42. Koelbel G, Schmiedl U, Griebel J *et al*. MR imaging of urinary bladder neoplasms. *J Comput Assist Tomogr* 1988; **12**: 98–103.

43. Maeda H, Kinukawa T, Hattori R *et al.* Detection of muscle layer invasion with submillimeter pixel MR images: staging of bladder carcinoma. *Magn Reson Imaging* 1995; **13**: 9–19.

44. Hayashi N, Tochigi H, Shiraishi T *et al.* A new staging criterion for bladder carcinoma using gadolinium-enhanced magnetic resonance imaging with an endorectal surface coil: a comparison with ultrasonography. *BJU Int* 2000; **85**: 32–6.

45. Takeda K, Kawaguchi T, Shiraishi T *et al.* Normal bladder wall morphology in Gd-DTPA-enhanced clinical MR imaging using an endorectal surface coil and histological assessment of submucosal linear enhancement using [14C]Gd-DOTA autoradiography in an animal model. *Eur J Radiol* 1998; **26**: 290–6.

46. Abu-Yousef M M, Narayana A S, Brown R C, Franken E A Jr. Urinary bladder tumors studied by cystosonography. Part II: Staging. *Radiology* 1984; **153**: 227–31.

47. Tsyb A F, Slesarev V I, Komarevtsev V N. Transvaginal longitudinal ultrasongraphy in diagnosis of carcinoma of the urinary bladder. *J Ultrasound Med* 1988; **7**: 179–82.

48. Karahan O I, Yikilmaz A, Ekmekcioglu O *et al.* Colour Doppler ultrasonography findings of bladder tumors: correlation with stage and histopathologic grade. *Acta Radiol* 2004; **25**: 481–6.

49. Horstman W G, McFarland R M, Gorman J D. Colour Doppler sonographic findings in patients with transitional cell carcinoma of the bladder and renal pelvis. *J Ultrasound Med* 1995; **14**: 129–33.

50. Akimoto T, Matsumoto M, Mitsuhashi N *et al.* Evaluation of effect of treatment for invasive bladder cancer by ultrasonography with intra-arterial infusion of carbon dioxide microbubbles. *Invest Radiol* 1997; **32**: 396–400.

51. Devonec M, Chapelon J Y, Codas H *et al.* Evaluation of bladder cancer with a miniature high frequency transurethral ultrasonography probe. *Br J Urol* 1987; **59**: 550–3.

52. Koraitim M, Kamal B, Metwalli N, Zaky Y. Transurethral ultrasonographic assessment of bladder carcinoma: its value and limitation. *J Urol* 1995; **154**: 375–8.

53. Saga Y, Numata A, Tokumitsu M *et al.* Comparative study of novel endoluminal ultrasonography and conventional transurethral ultrasonography in staging of bladder cancer. *Int J Urol* 2004; **11**: 597–601.

54. Grups J W, Gruss A, Frohmuller H G. Evaluation of the T stage carcinoma of the bladder by transurethral ultrasonography. *Urol Int* 1989; **44**: 132–4.

55. Jaeger N, Radeke H W, Adolphs H D *et al.* Value of intravesical sonography in tumor classification of bladder carcinoma. *Eur Urol* 1986; **12**: 76–84.

56. Holm H H, Juul N, Torp-Pedersen S *et al.* Bladder tumor staging by transurethral ultrasonic scanning. *Eur Urol* 1988; **15**: 31–3.

57. Hendrikx A J, Barentz J O, vd Stappen W A *et al.* The value of intravesical echography combined with double-surface coil magnetic resonnce imaging in staging bladder cancer. *Br J Urol* 1989; **63**: 469–75.

58. Horiuchi K, Tsuboi N, Shimizu H *et al.* High-frequency endoluminal ultrasonography for staging transitional cell carcinoma of the bladder. *Urology* 2000; **56**: 404–7.
59. Horiuchi K, Shimizu H, Yoshida K, Nishimura T. New ultrasonic cystofibrescope for staging bladder tumors. *J Endourol* 2005; **19**: 130–2.
60. Wagner B, Nesslauer T, Bartsch G Jr. *et al.* Staging bladder carcinoma by three-dimensional ultrasound rendering. *Ultrasound Med Biol* 2005; **31**: 301–5.
61. Ahlstrom H, Malmstrom P U, Letocha H *et al.* Positron emission tomography in the diagnosis and staging of urinary bladder cancer. *Acta Radiol* 1996; **37**: 180–5.
62. Letocha H, Ahlstrom H, Malmstrom P U *et al.* Positron emission tomography with L-methyl-11C-methionine in the monitoring of therapy response in muscle-invasive transitional cell carcinoma of the urinary bladder. *Br J Urol* 1994; **74**: 767–74.
63. Hara T, Kosaka N, Kondo T *et al.* Imaging of brain tumor, lung cancer, esophagus cancer, colon cancer, prostate cancer and bladder cancer with [C-11]choline. *J Nucl Med* 1997; **38**: 250p.
64. de Jong I J, Pruim J, Elsinga P H *et al.* Visualisation of bladder cancer using (11)C-choline PET: first clinical experience. *Eur J Nucl Med Mol Imaging* 2002; **29**: 1283–8.
65. Gofrit O N, Mishani E, Orevi M *et al.* Contribution of 11C-choline positron emission tomography/computerized tomography to preoperative staging of advanced transitional cell carcinoma. *J Urol* 2006; **176**: 940–4.
66. Picchio M, Treiber U, Beer A J *et al.* Value of 11C-choline PET and contrast-enhanced CT for staging of bladder cancer: correlation with histopathologic findings. *J Nucl Med* 2006; **47**: 938–44.
67. DeGrado T R, Coleman R E, Wang S *et al.* Synthesis and evaluation of 18F-labeled choline as an oncologic tracer for positron emission tomography: initial findings in prostate cancer. *Cancer Res* 2001; **61**: 110–17.
68. Simms M S, Perkins A C, Price M R *et al.* 99mTechnetium-C595 radioimmunoscintigraphy: a potential staging tool for bladder cancer. *BJU Int* 2001; **88**: 686–91.
69. Hughes O D, Perkins A C, Frier M *et al.* Imaging for staging bladder cancer: a clinical study of intravenous 111 indium-labelled anti-MUC1 mucin monoclonal antibody C595. *BJU Int* 2001; **87**: 39–46.

5

Imaging of metastatic bladder cancer

Jonathan Berry and David MacVicar

Introduction

In excess of 90% of tumors arising from the urinary bladder are urothelial carcinomas [1]. Alternative histological cell types which may rarely be encountered include squamous cell carcinoma, adenocarcinoma and tumors of mesenchymal origin.

Bladder cancer is a cause of significant morbidity and mortality throughout the world. Statistics demonstrate that between the years 2001 and 2003, 10 264 new cases of bladder cancer were diagnosed in the United Kingdom, and it was the seventh most common cause of malignancy-related death in males and eleventh most common cause in females [2]. Bladder cancer typically occurs in later life, with the peak incidence in the sixth and seventh decades. This, together with the strong association with environmental factors, likely accounts for the significant worldwide variation in incidence with, e.g. the incidence in the Italian male population being in excess of six times that in the Indian male population [3].

The prognosis of bladder cancer is dependent on a number of factors. Of particular importance are the depth of bladder wall invasion, the presence of metastases in lymph nodes and the presence of blood-borne metastases. In cases of superficial transitional cell malignancy, mean five-year survival of approximately 80% can be expected. Invasive tumors reduce five-year survival to less than 50%. If nodal metastases or blood-borne metastases are present then the five-year survival rate is worse still (15 and 5% respectively) [4,5]. Depending on local practice, up to one-third of patients may have metastatic disease at presentation [6]. Accurate assessment of both the primary tumor and the presence and extent of metastatic disease is therefore of paramount importance in prognostication and the optimal management of primary bladder malignancies.

Carcinoma of the Bladder, ed. David MacVicar. Published by Cambridge University Press. © Cambridge University Press 2008.

Patterns of metastatic bladder cancer

Historical data from autopsy series clearly demonstrates lymph nodes to be the most common site of metastatic disease, with an incidence of 78%. Other common sites of metastatic disease include the liver, lungs, bones and adrenals (Table 5.1) [7]. More recent studies based on computed tomography (CT) generally support this autopsy data [8]. It is the authors' experience that with the advent of widespread availability of cross-sectional imaging techniques, unusual sites of metastatic disease are being detected with increasing frequency.

Lymph node metastases

Lymph nodes are the most common site of metastatic disease. Whilst this fact has been known for some time, there has been ongoing debate regarding the extent of lymph node dissection required at the time of surgery for high-grade invasive bladder cancer. A more extensive nodal dissection potentially removes micrometastases and provides prognostic information, and this may allow modification of therapy but this remains controversial (see Chapter 6) [9–11]. Predicting which patients are likely to develop lymph node metastases would be of benefit in terms of both assessing prognosis and assigning appropriate management plans. Vascular endothelial growth factor (VEGF) is of importance in the angiogenesis and vasculogenesis of tumors. Early data suggests the expression of VEGF-C (a sub-type of VEGF) in biopsy samples is associated with the probability of a patient developing lymph node metastases [12]. Lymph node metastases occur initially in regional lymph nodes. The first groups involved include the anterior and lateral paravesical nodes, the lateral sacral nodes, and hypogastric, obturator and external iliac nodes.

Table 5.1. Sites of metastatic bladder cancer at autopsy [7]

Site	Incidence (%)
Lymph node	78
Liver	38
Lung	36
Bone	27
Adrenal gland	21
Intestine	13

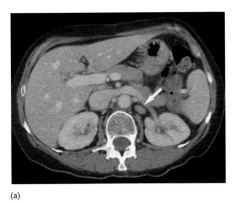
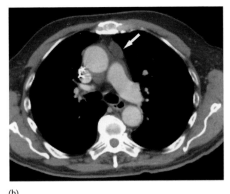

(a)   (b)

Figure 5.1 (a) Isolated left paraaortic lymph node metastasis (arrow) from a bladder urothelial malignancy. (b) Partially cystic anterior mediastinal lymph node enlargement (arrow). There is also a destructive metastasis within the body of the sternum.

Pathological nodes may subsequently be found in common iliac and paraaortic groups. Infiltrated nodes in the inguinal, mediastinal and cervical groups are less common (Fig. 5.1) [13–16].

Historically, bipedal lymphography has been used to assess metastatic disease within the pelvic and paraaortic lymph nodes. Although good accuracy rates for this technique have been reported, the procedure requires considerable expertise on the part of the operator and suffers from its inability to effectively demonstrate the obturator nodes [17,18]. Widespread availability of CT and MRI has resulted in bipedal lymphography now being rarely used.

Both CT and MRI assess nodal involvement on the basis of size. Unfortunately, while metastases from bladder cancer frequently infiltrate nodes, they commonly fail to cause significant nodal enlargement. Consequently, both CT and MRI assessments of lymph nodes are subject to a high false negative rate [19]. In addition, lymph node metastases from bladder cancer may enhance briskly following administration of intravenous contrast, making distinction of nodes from vascular structures difficult with CT [20] (Fig. 5.2a). Therefore, MRI may be of benefit when such doubt exists (Fig. 5.2b). It has been suggested that the degree of enhancement may be correlated to the aggressiveness of the tumor [4].

Benign nodes are typically oval in shape. When infiltrated, nodes tend to assume a more rounded shape. If, in addition to size, this morphological change is taken into consideration then nodes have been characterized as malignant with a sensitivity of 83% and a specificity of 98% [21]. Even using these two criteria there

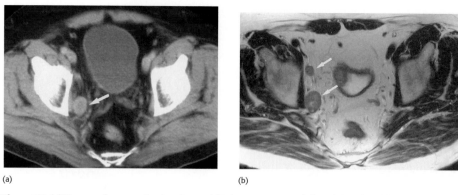

(a)   (b)

Figure 5.2 (a) Venous phase contrast-enhanced CT demonstrates a right pelvic sidewall structure (arrow) likely to represent a node showing intense peripheral enhancement following intravenous contrast. (b) Axial T2-weighted MRI confirms the presence of enlarged right pelvic sidewall lymph nodes (arrows).

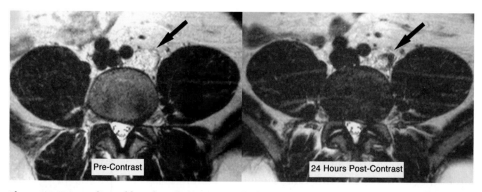

Figure 5.3 Retroperitoneal lymph node (arrows) at the level of the aortic bifurcation pre- and 24 hours post-administration of USPIO. A rim of low signal at the periphery of the node returns low signal as a result of ingestion of USPIO by macrophages in normal nodal tissue. In the remainder of the node, tumor has displaced macrophages and signal remains high on T2-weighted imaging.

remains the problem of detecting small morphologically normal nodes containing islands of malignant cells. There is evidence to suggest ultra-small superparamagnetic iron oxide particles (USPIO) may be of use in these circumstances. Following intravenous injection, USPIO are internalized by macrophages within lymph nodes. Imaging with a $T2^*$-weighted MR sequence reveals these iron-loaded lymph nodes to be of low signal. Tumor within a node of normal size and morphology replaces nodal tissue which contains macrophages. In the absence of macrophages to ingest the USPIO, tumor tissue will return intermediate or high signal, contrasting with low signal in normal nodal tissue (Fig. 5.3). Such a technique has been shown to significantly improve nodal staging in patients with bladder cancer with lymph nodes of normal size [22]. The drawbacks of this technique include the necessity to administer the contrast for over 30 minutes under medical supervision owing to the possibility of allergic reactions, and the fact that pre- and post-contrast imaging must be performed 24–36 hours apart.

Liver metastases

Although hepatic metastases are not uncommon in patients with disseminated bladder cancer, there is little data to suggest specific imaging features that enable bladder metastases to be distinguished from other hypovascular hepatic metastases. Hepatic metastases may be characterized using dynamic contrast-enhanced CT. When there is uncertainty regarding the interpretation of CT, MRI with or without contrast or occasionally positron emission tomography (PET)-CT may be employed (Fig. 5.4). Hepatic metastases are usually

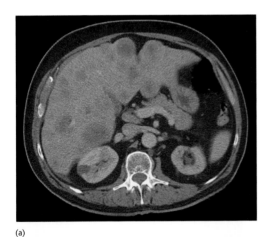

(a)

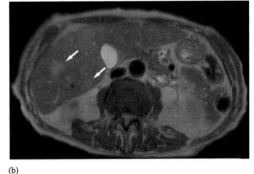

(b)

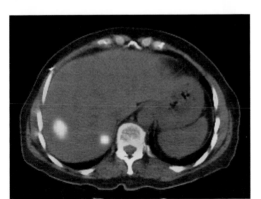

(c)

Figure 5.4 (a) Portal venous phase contrast-enhanced CT reveals numerous low attenuation metastases through all lobes of the liver in this patient known to have bladder cancer. (b) Axial T2-weighted MRI imaging of a different patient demonstrates several hyperintense lesions within the right liver (arrows). Percutaneous biopsy confirmed these to be hepatic metastases. (c) Fused axial FDG PET-CT images reveal avid FDG uptake within metabolically active metastases from urothelial neoplasm within the right lobe of the liver (see also color plate section).

multiple at the time of diagnosis and will often be associated with metastatic disease elsewhere. In circumstances when a liver lesion is found to be the sole site of metastatic disease, segmental hepatic resections have been successfully performed [23].

Lung metastases

As with liver metastases, lung metastases from a bladder primary typically occur late in the disease and are multiple at the time of diagnosis thus precluding surgical treatment options. However, lung metastases are occasionally the initial manifestation of metastatic disease from bladder cancer. Well-defined pulmonary nodules may be seen on a chest radiograph but are most accurately assessed with CT (Fig. 5.5). Cavitating or spiculated lesions are unusual, but lung metastases from urothelial malignancy may take virtually any form.

Bone metastases

Bone metastases resulting from a primary bladder tumor are most commonly osteoblastic in nature and therefore result in sclerotic bone lesions. Less commonly, osteolytic lesions may be seen. Plain radiographs, CT, MRI, PET-CT and bone

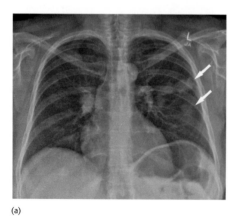
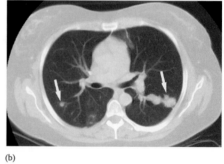

(a)   (b)

Figure 5.5 (a) Routine follow-up chest radiograph in a patient who had previously undergone treatment for invasive urothelial malignancy reveals numerous soft tissue density nodules within both lungs (arrows). (b) Axial CT confirms the presence of widespread pulmonary metastases (arrows).

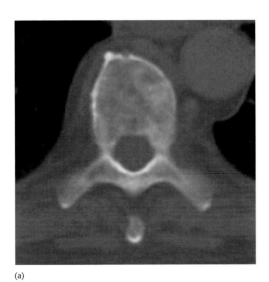

(a)

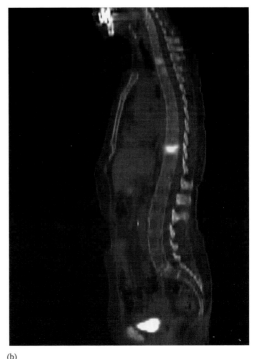

(b)

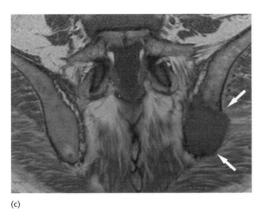

(c)

Figure 5.6 (a) Targeted axial CT image of a thoracic vertebra in a patient with bladder malignancy demonstrates ill-defined mixed lytic and sclerotic lesions in the vertebral body. (b) Fused sagittal FDG PET-CT confirms the presence of metabolically active metastases within the vertebrae (see also color plate section). (c) Coronal T1-weighted MRI reveals expansile low signal metastasis centred on the left iliac bone (arrows).

scintigraphy may be used in isolation or combination in the detection of bone metastases (Fig. 5.6).

Studies have indicated the vertebrae and pelvic bones to be the most common sites of metastatic bone disease although almost any bone may be involved (Table 5.2) [24]. Relative to disease within the lymph nodes or lungs, bone metastases typically respond poorly to chemotherapeutic agents [25]. Even so, there are reported cases of

Table 5.2. Anatomical distribution of bone metastasis arising from primary urothelial tumor, as established by radiographic studies [24]

Site	Percentage
Spine	40
Pelvis	26
Femur	10
Ribs	10
Humerus	5
Tibia	3
Skull	2
Clavicle	2
Mandible	1
Sternum	1

patients with advanced metastatic bone disease achieving complete response following chemotherapy, although these are exceptional [26].

Uncommon sites of metastatic disease

There are a variety of unusual sites of metastatic disease reported in the literature. Whilst some of these, such as metastatic deposits in the soft tissues of the hand [27], are extremely rare and have only limited number of case reports, others are more widely reported.

Cutaneous metastatic deposits from primary bladder cancer occurs in only 0.84–3.6% of patients and usually represents a poor prognostic sign, with a median disease-specific survival of less than 12 months from time of diagnosis [28]. Whilst some cutaneous deposits may be related to iatrogenic implantation following instrumentation or surgery, many of the documented locations of deposits are not compatible with this mode of spread [29]. Both systemic chemotherapy and local electrochemotherapy have been used in the treatment of these lesions [30].

Ocular metastases are most commonly associated with primary malignancies of the breast, lung and stomach. There are a few case reports documenting this as a site of metastatic disease from primary bladder cancer. In such cases, ocular metastasis may present with a range of signs and symptoms, including proptosis, diplopia and pain. Mode of spread to the eye is via the hematogenous route, with choroidal and orbital sites being the most common locations [31]. Whilst both ultrasound and CT may be used to visualize these deposits, MRI, including fat-saturated sequences, are likely to provide the most accurate anatomical definition. Both systemic chemotherapy and local radiotherapy have been employed in the treatment of ocular metastases with limited effect.

Approximately 300 cases of penile metastases from all known primaries have been documented in the literature worldwide, of which at least 73 were from a bladder malignancy. These lesions are frequently located within the shaft of the penis and as such are amenable to examination by ultrasound and, if required, MRI. Given the location of these lesions, direct spread of tumor from the primary site is unlikely although some authors have suggested iatrogenic spread following transurethral procedures. An alternative possibility is hematogenous spread via the penile venous system that communicates with the venous plexus of the bladder and prostate [32]. Regardless of mode of spread and method of diagnosis, historical data suggests survival after diagnosis of penile metastasis is only approximately 3.9 months [33].

Central nervous system (CNS) metastases from bladder malignancy are traditionally thought of as rare. However, with increasing effective chemotherapeutics, metastases to the "sanctuary sites" such as the CNS are more commonly being found. Of the CNS metastases, intra-parenchymal brain metastases are the most common and are well visualized on post-contrast CT or MRI (Fig. 5.7). Less common is the finding of meningeal metastases [34]. Meningeal nodularity and enhancement is often difficult to appreciate with contrast-enhanced CT and is most easily detected with gadolinium-enhanced MRI in axial and coronal planes.

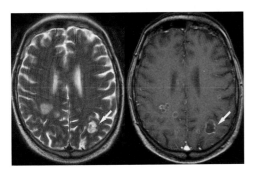

Figure 5.7 In this patient with bladder cancer axial T2-weighted (left) and gadolinium enhanced T1-weighted (right) MRI images of the brain demonstrate numerous T2 high-signal, peripherally enhancing intra-axial metastases within both cerebral hemispheres.

Imaging follow-up of bladder cancer

Imaging follow-up and re-staging following treatment of bladder cancer remains controversial and may on occasion be technically challenging owing to the distortion of normal anatomy resulting from previous intervention [35]. In one study, in the absence of abnormal clinical signs or symptoms, CT alone detected only 10% of recurrences [36]. On the basis of this finding, some advocate that imaging follow-up of treated bladder cancer is not warranted, and cystoscopic surveillance alone is indicated.

Those who support follow-up imaging state the aim is to detect recurrent or metastatic disease and, given the epidemiological factors predisposing to bladder cancer commonly result in "field effect", to detect "new"/previously unseen tumors. The risk of recurrent disease or metastatic disease depends on a number of factors including whether the original tumor invasion was superficial or deep, the size of the original tumor and the grade of malignancy [37]. Of these factors, the depth of tumor invasion is most important.

For superficial tumors, the risk of a second malignancy arising at a later date is probably greater than the risk of recurrence or metastasis from a treated tumor. Therefore, some suggest screening of both the urinary bladder and upper renal tracts is appropriate. Historically, this has been achieved using intravenous urography (IVU). Increasingly, CT urography (CTU) and more recently MR urography (MRU) are being employed. Although often more expensive than IVU, these provide the advantages of accurate anatomical delineation, assessment of extra-luminal disease and, in the case of MR urography, negate the need to use iodinated contrast media. In terms of frequency and duration of screening, some authors suggest a single baseline study is all that is required, while others advocate imaging every 6 or 12 months for anything from two years to life [38].

Support for follow-up of invasive bladder cancer is stronger although a consensus as to what is appropriate follow-up has not yet been reached. Most suggested follow-up programs are based upon, either in isolation or combination, chest radiography, investigation of the upper renal tracts (using IVU, CTU or MRU) and CT or MRI to image the abdomen and pelvis. The suggested frequency and duration of these investigations vary between authors. Current American College of Radiology guidelines [37] recommend patients with invasive cancer have investigation of the upper renal tracts every one to two years. In addition, those patients with invasive cancer requiring cystectomy should have an MRI or CT at 6, 12 and 24 months and a chest radiograph at 6, 12, 18, 24, 36, 48 and 60 months post-operatively.

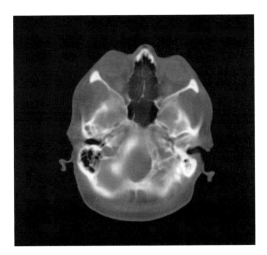

Figure 5.8 In a patient with known metastatic urothelial cancer to the liver and bones, fused axial FDG PET-CT demonstrates avid FDG uptake within a radiographically occult metastasis within the right skull base to be the cause for the patient's symptoms (see also color plate section).

At present, PET is not routinely employed in the staging or follow-up of bladder cancer. Although there are some studies which support its use, it has not gained widespread support [39,40]. Flurodeoxyglucose (FDG) is subject to urinary excretion and therefore high levels of activity are normally found within the bladder. As a result, distinguishing normal bladder activity from tumor and regional spread or nodes has been difficult. The advent of PET-CT has resulted in improved delineation of anatomical structures relative to sites of activity and is therefore likely to be beneficial in the imaging of bladder cancer. Certainly, PET-CT is on occasion a useful problem-solving tool in the assessment of metastatic disease (Fig. 5.8). Future developments in this field may include the use of ^{11}C-methionine as an alternative tracer to FDG although at present limited access to this radiopharmaceutical prevents its widespread use.

Conclusion

As with most solid tumors, bladder cancer usually spreads first to local lymph nodes but virtually any organ is involved in advanced metastatic disease. Consensus on the usefulness of imaging surveillance strategies has not been reached, although the American College of Radiology guidelines [37] represent an attempt to clarify the situation. The presence of metastatic disease adversely affects prognosis and in these circumstances imaging choices are influenced by clinical goals of prognostication and palliation.

REFERENCES

1. Wong-You-Cheong J J, Woodward P J, Manning M A, Sesterhenn I A. From the archives of the AFIP: neoplasms of the urinary bladder: radiologic-pathologic correlation. *Radiographics* 2006; **26**(2): 553–80.

2. Office of National Statistics. Cancer incidence and mortality in the United Kingdom 2001–03. http://www.statistics.gov.uk/statbase/Product.asp?vlnk=14209.

3. Kirkali Z, Chan T, Manoharan M *et al.* Bladder cancer: epidemiology, staging and grading, and diagnosis. *Urology* 2005; **66**(6 suppl 1): 4–34.

4. Crawford E D, Wood D P, Petrylak D P *et al.* Southwest oncology group studies in bladder cancer. *Cancer* 2003; **97**: 2099–108.

5. de Wit R. European Organization for Research and Treatment. Overview of bladder cancer trials in the European Organization for Research and Treatment. *Cancer* 2003; **97**(8 suppl): 2120–6.

6. Raghavan D. *The Management of Bladder Cancer.* London: Edward Arnold, 1988.

7. Babaian R J, Johnson D E, Llamas L, Ayala A G. Metastases from transitional cell carcinoma of urinary bladder. *Urology* 1980; **16**(2): 142–4.

8. Hassan J M, Cookson M S, Smith J A Jr., Chang S S. Patterns of initial transitional cell recurrence in patients after cystectomy. *J Urol* 2006; **175**(6): 2054–7.

9. Stein J P. Lymphadenectomy in bladder cancer: how high is "high enough". *Urol Oncol* 2006; **24**(4): 349–55.

10. Liedberg F, Mansson W. Lymph node metastasis in bladder cancer. *Eur Urol* 2006; **49**(1): 13–21.

11. Hoshi S, Orikasa S, Suzuki K I *et al.* Diagnosis and treatment of pelvic lymph node metastasis in bladder control. *Int J Urol* 1999; **6**(8): 400–7.

12. Zu X, Tang Z, Li Y *et al.* Vascular endothelial growth factor-C expression in bladder transitional cell cancer and its relationship to lymph node metastasis. *BJU Int* 2006; **98**(5): 1090–3.

13. Husband J E. Staging bladder cancer. *Clin Radiol* 1992; **46**(3): 153–9.

14. Mead G M, Roberts J T. The role of the nonsurgical oncologist in the management of advanced transitional cell cancer. Part II: metastatic disease. *BJU Int* 2004; **94**(7): 981–4.

15. Park J M, Charnsangavej C, Yoshimitsu K *et al.* Pathways of nodal metastasis from pelvic tumors: CT demonstration. *Radiographics* 1994; **14**(6): 1309–21.

16. Husband J E, Koh D-M. Bladder cancer. In: Husband J E, Reznek R H, eds. *Imaging in Onclogy,* (2nd edn). London: Taylor Francis, 2004.

17. Chagnon S, Cochand-Priollet B, Gzaeil M *et al.* Pelvic cancers: staging of 139 cases with lymphography and fine-needle aspiration biopsy. *Radiology* 1989; **173**(1): 103–6.

18. Wajsman Z, Baumgartner G, Murphy G P, Merrin C. Evaluation of lymphangiography for clinical staging of bladder tumors. *J Urol* 1975; **114**(5): 712–14.

19. Koss J C, Arger P H, Coleman B G, Mulhern *et al.* CT staging of bladder carcinoma. *AJR Am J Roentgenol* 1981; **137**(2): 359–62.

20. Husband J E, Robinson L, Thomas G. Contrast enhancing lymph nodes in bladder cancer: a potential pitfall on CT. *Clin Radiol* 1992; **45**(6): 395–8.

21 Jager G J, Barentsz, J O, Oosterhof G O *et al.* Pelvic adenopathy in prostatic and urinary bladder carcinoma: MR imaging with a three-dimensional TI-weighted magnetization-prepared-rapid gradient-echo sequence. *AJR Am J Roentgenol* 1996; **167**(6): 1503–7.

22. Deserno W M, Harisinghani M G, Taupitz M *et al.* Urinary bladder cancer: preoperative nodal staging with ferumoxtran-10-enhanced MR imaging. *Radiology* 2004; **233**(2): 449–56.

23. Gallagher H J, Redmond H P, Deasy J, McLean P A. Hepatic resection of solitary metastasis from transitional cell carcinoma of the bladder. *J Urol* 1998; **159**(3): 986.

24. Sengelov L, Kamby C, von der Maase H. Pattern of metastases in relation to characteristics of primary tumor and treatment in patients with disseminated urothelial carcinoma. *J Urol* 1996; **155**(1): 111–14.

25. Sternberg C N, Yagoda A, Scher H I *et al.* (1988). M-VAC (methotrexate, vinblastine, doxorubicin and cisplatin) for advanced transitional cell carcinoma of the urothelium. *J Urol* 1988; **139**(3): 461–9.

26. Joudi F N, Dahmoush L, Spector D M, Konety B R. Complete response of bony metastatic bladder urothelial cancer to neoadjuvant chemotherapy and cystectomy. *Urol Oncol* 2006; **24**(5): 403–6.

27. Heymans M, Jardon-Jeghers C, Vanwijck R. Hand metastases from urothelial tumor. *J Hand Surg [Am]* 1990; **15**(3): 509–11.

28. Block C A, Dahmoush L, Konety B R. Cutaneous metastases from transitional cell carcinoma of the bladder. *Urology* 2006; **67**(4): 846.e15–17.

29. Akman Y, Cam K, Kavak A, Alper M. Extensive cutaneous metastasis of transitional cell carcinoma of the bladder. *Int J Urol* 2003; **10**(2): 103–4.

30. Kubota Y, Mir L M, Nakada T *et al.* Successful treatment of metastatic skin lesions with electrochemotherapy. *J Urol* 1998; **160**(4): 1426.

31. Nabi G, Dadeya S, Dogra P N, Lal H. Eye metastasis form urothelial tumours. *Int Urol Nephrol* 2002; **34**(1): 51–4.

32. Berger A P, Rogatsch H, Hoeltl L *et al.* Late penile metastasis from primary bladder carcinoma. *Urology* 2003; **62**(1): 145.

33. Haddad F S. Penile metastases secondary to bladder cancer. Review of the literature. *Urol Int* 1984; **39**(3): 125–42.

34. Eng C, Cunningham D, Quade B J *et al.* Meningeal carcinomatosis from transitional cell carcinoma of the bladder. *Cancer* 1993; **72**(2): 553–7.

35. MacVicar A D. Bladder cancer staging. *BJU Int* 2000; **86** (suppl 1): 111–22.

36. Slaton J W, Swanson D A, Grossman H B, Dinney C P. A stage specific approach to tumor surveillance after radical cystectomy for transitional cell carcinoma of the bladder. *J Urol* 1999; **162**(3 Pt 1): 710–14.

37. American College of Radiology Appropriateness Criteria–Follow-up Imaging of Bladder Carcinoma (2003) http://www.acr.org/s_acr/bin.asp?TrackID=&SID=1&DID=11840&CID=1202&VID=2&DOC=File.PDF

38. Bradford T J, Montie J E, Hafez K S. The role of imaging in the surveillance of urologic malignancies. *Urol Clin North Am* 2006; **33**(3): 377–96.

39. Kosuda S, Kison P V, Greenough R *et al.* Preliminary assessment of fluorine-18 fluorodeoxyglucose positron emission tomography in patients with bladder cancer. *Eur J Nucl Med* 1997; **24**(6): 615–20.

40. Drieskens O, Oyen R, Van Poppel H *et al.* FDG-PET for preoperative staging of bladder cancer. *Eur J Nucl Med Mol Imaging* 2005; **32**(12): 1412–17.

6

Surgery for bladder cancer

Sarb Sandhu and Alan Thompson

Introduction

The majority of patients (approx 70%) who present with bladder cancer have superficial disease. Thirty percent of these patients will progress to muscle invasive disease. The remaining patients will present with disease that is already invading the muscle (pT2 – 4) or metastatic. The surgical management of these two types of disease is distinct. The principle objective when treating patients with superficial disease is to prevent progression, the secondary objective is to prevent recurrence. The primary aim in the management of patients with muscle invasive disease confined to the bladder is to prevent further progression and so if a cystectomy is undertaken the aim is oncological cure.

Transurethral resection of bladder cancer

The diagnosis of bladder cancer is based on examination of the histological specimen obtained by transurethral resection. In patients with superficial disease the tumor, along with bladder wall, including some muscle is resected. This allows the histopathologist to accurately stage the patient and if the tumor has been completely resected with clear margins, treatment may be considered adequate and the patient will commence follow-up or surveillance.

In patients proved to have muscle invasive disease at histology, transurethral resection should be considered a diagnostic procedure only. Random biopsies are not usually indicated but areas suspicious for carcinoma should be biopsied. Patients with muscle invasive bladder cancer can be treated with either radical radiotherapy or cystectomy. The choice of which modality to use depends in the main upon the views of the patient, but there are a few relative indications

Carcinoma of the Bladder, ed. David MacVicar. Published by Cambridge University Press. © Cambridge University Press 2008.

for surgery. These are intractable bleeding, a small-capacity bladder, severe dysuria and ureteric obstruction. The use of neoadjuvant chemotherapy has been advocated by some authors in conjunction with both of these treatment options (see Chapter 8).

Techniques for surgical management of muscle invasive bladder cancer

Cystectomy

Radical cystoprostatectomy in the male patient and anterior exenteration in the female patient, coupled with en bloc pelvic lymphadenectomy, remain the standard surgical approaches to muscle invasive bladder cancer in the absence of metastatic disease. Patients should be offered cystectomy only if the disease is confined to the bladder. The presence of metastatic disease is considered a contraindication for curative cystectomy. The aim of radical cystectomy is to obtain oncological cure with minimal morbidity. Patients who are candidates for radical cystectomy should have preoperative staging; this includes pathological staging of the bladder cancer, clinical staging with bimanual examination under anesthetic and radiological staging.

If reconstruction is being advocated, patients should have a glomerular filtration rate (GFR) above 40 ml/min and the type of reconstruction will be determined by the pathology. Male patients in whom an orthotopic reconstruction is being considered should not have disease involving the urethra and ideally not involving the prostate. In female patients disease involving the bladder neck and trigone should also preclude an orthotopic reconstruction. The presence of multifocal CIS is also a relative contraindication to an orthotopic reconstruction. Patients who are being offered orthotopic reconstruction should not have had previous urethral surgery, and a history of urethral strictures or incontinence is also a relative contraindication. Patients should be carefully counseled about the risks of incontinence and some may even need to perform intermittent self-catheterization after surgery.

Patients not suitable for an orthotopic reconstruction can be offered a continent Mainz pouch or a continent cutaneous pouch. The alternative is an ileal conduit. All of these techniques are discussed in greater detail later.

Patients should undergo adequate bowel preparation using appropriate purgatives the day prior to surgery. They should be well hydrated, have cross-matched blood available, and undertake measures to prevent deep vein thrombosis, which may include thromboembolic deterrent stockings, flotron boots and subcutaneous heparin.

The standard cystectomy in the male is performed using the transperitoneal approach. Once the peritoneum is entered via a lower midline incision, the urachus is mobilized. The peritoneal cavity is inspected to ensure there is no macroscopic evidence of metastases. Bilateral pelvic lymphadenectomy is performed. The landmarks for a standard lymphadenectomy are cephalad, the bifurcation of the iliac vessels, and caudally, the endopelvic fascia. The lateral landmark is the genitofemoral nerve, and the medial, the obturator nerve. Every attempt should be made to ligate or seal the lymphatic channels with either an energy source or mechanically with liga-clips. The latter have the advantage of being radioopaque and therefore demarcate the extent of the dissection, thus allowing post-operative assessment and planning of adjuvant radiotherapy.

The vascular blood supply to the bladder is from a number of sources and the arterial and venous anatomy are variable. The superior and inferior vesical pedicles arise from the internal iliac vessels and are ligated and divided. Once these are divided, the rectovesical cul-de-sac is entered in the male and the peritoneum divided below the insertion of the ureters. In the male the vas is identified and divided. The ureters are then clipped in continuity and divided. It is important that there is no urine leakage from the bladder at this stage of the procedure. The tips of the ureters can be sent for frozen section analysis if required. The bladder and prostate are carefully dissected off the rectum. As dissection proceeds caudally, the endopelvic fascia is identified and incised. This allows better visualization of the vascular pedicles of the prostate, which are identified, ligated and divided. Four anterior structures, the puboprostatic (or pubovesical) ligaments, the dorsal vein complex of Santorini, the membranous urethra and the rectourethralis, remain to be divided. The puboprostatic ligaments are divided under direct vision. A number of strategies have been proposed to control the dorsal vein complex: Some surgeons pass a right-angled clamp under this complex and tie it in continuity, others recommend using a babcock, and some divide it and over-sew the open ends. Whichever strategy is chosen, control is essential. If control of this complex is not established, life-threatening hemorrhage can ensue. Furthermore, good views of the urethra are essential if an orthotopic reconstruction is to be undertaken. The urethra and the rectourethralis are then divided and the specimen is removed.

In the female, the supporting ligaments may need to be divided, and an anterior strip of vagina is removed in continuity with the bladder, and unless the urethra is required for reconstruction this is also removed. The vaginal remnant can be closed in either the vertical plane, or if the patient is sexually active a posterior anterior closure may give better functional results. To complete the anterior exenteration, the uterus, fallopian tubes, and ovaries should be removed; however, in modern practice there is often no need to remove these structures unless clinically indicated.

It is mandatory at all stages of this operation that urine that has been in contact with cancer must not be allowed to contaminate the operative field.

The overall five-year disease-free survival, following radical removal of the bladder, is between 48 and 68%. This is clearly dependent upon stage, with patients with pT1 disease having reported five-year disease-free survival rates of 75–83%, pT2 of 63–89%, pT3 of 31–78%, and pT4 of 21–50%. The majority of patients who are disease free at five years remain disease free long-term [1–3].

Nerve-sparing cystectomy

The advent of orthotopic reconstruction, and better immediate surgical outcomes, has led to an increasing focus on the long-term morbidity associated with pelvic surgery. In the male patient, impotence has been traditionally regarded as an acceptable consequence of radical cystectomy. However, better understanding of the anatomy of the nerves responsible for potency has allowed prevention of this complication.

In young children, the prostate is a small structure, and the nervii erigentes run from the plexus on the rectum to the base of the seminal vesicles and encase the prostate [4]. The accepted wisdom has been that as the prostate grows, the nerves are pushed posteriorly and form a distinct band, which accompanies the vascular supply and forms the neurovascular bundles of the penis. Recent work has questioned this view. The newer paradigm is that as the prostate grows, the nerves are stretched and encase the prostate, and the whole of the prostatic fascia has these nerves running through it [4]. Therefore, in order to achieve a nerve-sparing cystectomy, a retrograde approach starting at the apex of the prostate has been advocated. The puboprostatic ligaments are divided and the prostate fascia is carefully dissected off the prostate. Santorini's plexus is divided, the apex of the prostate is transected and the rectourethralis is divided. The prostate is then removed in a retrograde fashion. At all times diathermy should be avoided.

Once this step is completed, a standard antegrade cystectomy is performed until one reaches the seminal vesicles. At this stage, the tips of the seminal vesicles are preserved if possible. Once the cystoprostatectomy specimen has been removed, reconstruction can be undertaken if appropriate.

Using these and other techniques it is possible to achieve potency in 70–80% of men undergoing cystoprostatectomy [5,6].

Vagina-sparing cystectomy

In the female patient, the anterior vaginal wall is often excised with the main specimen. If, however, in a sexually active patient this can be preserved without an adverse oncological outcome [7], it may lead to preservation of sexual function. The lymphatic drainage of the bladder base and the trigone occurs along the lateral vaginal wall, and so if vaginal preservation is to be attempted, these areas must be free of tumor [8].

The autonomic nerves which provide the urethral sphincter with tonic activity and the vaginal glands with stimulation run along the postero-lateral aspect of the vagina. Therefore, by carefully dissecting the bladder off the anterior vaginal wall these can be preserved. The cystectomy can then be performed, preserving as much urethral length as possible if an orthotopic reconstruction is to be undertaken.

In a carefully selected population of patients, a successful functional outcome can be achieved [9]. The short-term data regarding the preservation of sexual function is encouraging [10], but as yet there is no long-term data.

Management of the male urethra

Historically, prophylactic urethrectomy was carried out with radical cystectomy. However, this precludes the option of orthotopic reconstruction, and also adds to the surgical morbidity associated with this procedure.

Most surgeons are prepared to leave the urethra *in situ* provided there is no evidence of carcinoma in the region of the trigone or the bladder neck, the prostatic fossa or the urethra itself. In our experience, this decreases the morbidity of this procedure, and, if coupled with a nerve-sparing cystectomy, leads to a greater number of men preserving their potency.

Management of the female urethra

Urethrectomy in the female patient does not add to the morbidity of the procedure. Therefore patients who are not having an orthotopic reconstruction should have a simultaneous urethrectomy.

The presence of tumor involving the urethra or bladder neck is a contraindication to urethra-preserving surgery.

Prostate-sparing cystectomy

Nerve-sparing radical prostatectomy can lead to improvements in sexual function after radical cystectomy. Further improvements can be achieved if prostatectomy is avoided. Patients may be able to experience ejaculation (retrograde) as well as being potent and so be able to experience a more complete orgasm.

If prostate-sparing surgery is advocated, it is important to make sure that there is no evidence of prostate cancer, and if necessary, biopsies should be taken to maximize the certainty that coexistent prostatic carcinoma is not present. The patient's bladder cancer should be remote from the prostatic urethra. In addition, since most orthotopic reservoirs are low-pressure systems, the patient will need to have transurethral resection of the prostate prior to reconstruction.

If prostate-sparing cystectomy is undertaken with orthotopic reconstruction, day-time continence rates in excess of 95% can be achieved, with potency rates of between 70% and 80% [11,12].

Partial cystectomy

Partial cystectomy involves removal of a full-thickness segment of the bladder wall, which includes a tumor. A margin of 1–2 cm is usually preserved. The bladder is then reconstructed. The patient must have an adequate bladder capacity for this treatment.

The role of partial cystectomy in treatment of primary vesical disease is limited to patients with TCC within a diverticulum, or adenocarcinoma of the urachus. In rare circumstances, it can be performed in patients with a solitary focus of muscle invasive TCC; however, this is not standard treatment.

Partial cystectomy is also mainly used when the bladder is involved by direct invasion of a tumor from a neighbouring organ. A segment of bladder with an adequate clearance margin can be taken and the bladder reconstructed. Care must be taken to prevent the ureters from being damaged, which if necessary should be protected with ureteric stents.

Salvage cystectomy

Salvage cystectomy is undertaken in patients who have recurrence after treatment with radical radiotherapy. The steps of the surgical procedure are identical to a standard cystectomy, but due to the effects of radiotherapy these operations can be a technical challenge. The desmoplastic reaction caused by radiotherapy can lead to difficulty in identifying anatomical planes and so sharp dissection is often required. In addition, there is an increased risk of intestinal complications, with one series reporting a 8.7% bowel leakage rate after salvage cystectomy [13].

Orthotopic reconstruction after salvage cystectomy has been undertaken with acceptable results [14]. Only limited data is available on the outcomes in patients who had undergone salvage cystectomy; the overall reported five-year survival is 5–45% depending in part upon the stage of the disease and the initial response to radiotherapy.

Pelvic lymphadenectomy

The role of lymphadenectomy in the surgical management of muscle invasive bladder cancer is a point of contention. Is the role of lymphadenectomy to provide additional staging information or to cure patients with disease that has metastasized to a limited number of regional nodes? Anatomical studies by Ghoneim's group in Egypt have identified the sentinel node-bearing region as the endopelvic region, between the internal iliac and obturator group of nodes [15]. In 22 patients with single node involvement who had undergone extended lymphadenectomy, the involved node was identified in the sentinel region in 21 cases. There were no skip lesions and they concluded that although bilateral pelvic node dissection was mandatory, negative nodes in the sentinel region indicated that more proximal dissection was not required.

At the time of cystectomy, 25% of patients have lymph node involvement. The overall five-year survival of patients with node positive disease is 40%. This is influenced by the number of nodes involved and the pathological stage of the primary cancer [16]. The five-year survival of patients with pT2N1 disease is good and approximates to that of pT2N0 disease; the survival of patients with extrapelvic nodal disease beyond the region of the endopelvic fascia is poor, and so extensive dissection may not be of any benefit [17].

Complications of radical cystectomy

In the UK, peri-operative and 30-day mortality has almost been eradicated. The National Institute for Clinical Excellence have proposed that all major cancer centers performing cystectomy should have a mortality of less than 4% associated with this operation. The overall complication rate following radical cystectomy is approximately 25%. The peri-operative complications relate to blood loss and damage to adjacent viscera. Wound complications may occur and tend to be related to body mass index and nutritional status. Gastrointestinal complications include intestinal obstruction, fistula, leakage of intestinal contents and rectal injury. Post-operatively, early mobilization should be encouraged to prevent and treat pulmonary atelectasis and other respiratory complications, as well as preventing deep vein thrombosis and pulmonary emboli.

Other complications relate to uretero-intestinal anastomosis, where there can be leakage of urine and stenosis, or relate to sexual dysfunction. Some of these complications are managed by radiological techniques; patients with urinary leaks often require image-guided insertion of tube drains, reinsertion of ureteric stents percutaneously and occasionally nephrostomies. Patients with uretero-ileal stenosis are candidates for antegrade balloon dilation of the stricture and insertion of stents.

Urinary diversion

After a cystectomy has been performed, the urine has to be diverted. The options that exist at present are an ileal conduit, an orthotopic neobladder, a ureterosigmoidostomy (Mainz 2) or a cutaneous continent pouch.

Ileal conduit

The ileal conduit is a long-established form of urinary diversion. Avoiding the terminal ileum for metabolic reasons, 10–15 cm of distal ileum is mobilized and isolated on its vascular pedicle. The isolated segment of bowel is placed caudally and an ileo-ileal anastomosis is performed to reinstate continuity of the remainder of the small bowel. The mesenteric window is closed to prevent hernia formation.

Traditionally, the ileal conduit is placed on the right side of the abdominal wall. In such cases, the left ureter is mobilized and is brought to the right side of the abdomen below the sigmoid mesentery and above the great vessels. The ureters can be anastomosed to the ileum separately (Bricker technique) or the terminal ends anastomosed to each other to form a ureteric plate, which is then anastomosed to the proximal end of the ileal segment (Wallace technique). The Bricker anastomosis is an end-to-side anastomosis. The advantage of this technique is that if there is tumor recurrence in one ureter there is no direct physical channel for the contralateral ureter to become involved. The disadvantage of the Bricker technique is the anastomotic stricture rate of approximately 7%, which is twice the stricture rate of a Wallace anastomosis. Both types of anastomoses are refluxing and both anastomoses are protected by stents for 10–14 days. It is important to anastomose all of the ureters to the bowel segment; this is particularly pertinent in patients with duplex ureters.

The distal end of the ileum is brought to the surface at a predetermined position. The ileal conduit should traverse the rectus sheath, and the stoma should not be flush but be protruding. In obese patients, it is often difficult to form an end stoma, and a loop ileostomy (Turnbull) may be easier.

The complications of an ileal conduit include prolapse, necrosis, parastomal herniation, obstruction, dermatitis, stomal stenosis and calculi. Those complications related to the uretero-ileal anastomosis include urinary leakage, recurrent urinary infections, stenosis and obstruction and upper tract deterioration. The complications related to an ileal conduit are ongoing, with 94% of patients surviving more than 15 years having some complications. Of particular concern are upper tract dilation and the accompanied loss of renal function [18,19].

Although rarely used, other segments of bowel have been used to form conduits, including the colon and the jejunum. Some surgeons perform tunneled ureteric anastomosis in an attempt to prevent reflux, but this increases the risk of stricture formation and also makes endoscopic surveillance of the upper tracts difficult.

Orthotopic reconstruction

Orthotopic reconstruction involves the use of the patient's native urethra as an outlet, and their urethral sphincter as the continence mechanism. A number of different types of reservoir have been advocated. All require a segment of bowel, which is detubularized. The bowel is detubularized to form a plate, which is then folded over, and the bowel segment is reconfigured into a sphere. This has two main advantages: For a given length of bowel this allows the volume to be increased by 50%, and secondly it converts the segment from a high pressure system with peristaltic waves into a low pressure reservoir with limited motor activity and so potentially decreasing the risk of incontinence. Although the literature supports the first conclusion, the second is still debated.

Small bowel reservoirs

The commonest reservoir used in clinical practice is the Studer J-reservoir. This is constructed from 50 to 60 cm of ileum. The distal 35–40 cm of ileum is detubularized and reconfigured into a sphere, and this is anastomosed to the urethra. The ureters are anastomosed into the proximal isoperistaltic limb of the J. This is a low-pressure system and voiding is by the voluntary relaxation of the external sphincter and performing a Valsalva maneuver. This results in almost complete emptying without reflux.

Long-term follow-up data available from the Bern group in men found that at ten years the day-time continence rate was 91% while the night-time continence rate was 60%. In 96% of cases there was no significant loss in renal parenchymal thickness. After ten years only one patient had post-void residual volume of greater than 100 ml. The reservoir capacity increased to a maximum at 12 months (mean capacity = 462 ml) and was stable for up to five years and decreased slightly thereafter [20].

Promising results have also been obtained with this procedure in female patients [9].

The Hautman W is another orthotopic reservoir that is often used: 40–60 cm of small bowel is used, the bowel is then arranged as a W, opened along its anti-mesenteric border and a detubularized sphere is reconstructed. The ureters are then usually placed in serous-lined extramural tunnels. Results from Hautmann's group in Ulm, Germany, and Ghoneim's group in Mansoura, Egypt, have shown that this is an effective reconstruction [21,22].

Large bowel reservoirs

Detubularized segments of large bowel have also been used as orthotopic reservoirs; the principles are the same as for small bowel reservoir, except that 20 cm of large bowel is usually adequate. Follow-up for these reservoirs is limited, but initial reports are promising.

Ureterosigmoidostomy

The traditional ureterosigmoidostomy consisted of anastomosing the ureters to the sigmoid and using the anal sphincter as the continence mechanism. However, this procedure led to rapid renal deterioration, ascending infections, poor continence, and metabolic disturbances. This procedure was therefore abandoned. By applying the principles of detubularization and the serous-lined extramural tunnel, the group from Mainz resurrected this technique, with good results.

The Mainz 2 ureterosigmoidostomy can be used in patients who do not have a functioning urethral sphincter or urethra: 30–36 cm of sigmoid colon is positioned in an S-shape, the bowel is opened along its anti-mesenteric border and reconfigured as a sphere, and the ureters are placed in serous extramural tunnels and anchored in the reservoir. Ten-year follow-up data is available and 97% continence is reported. Over the same period there was a 7% ureteric implantation stenosis, while 70% of the patients required oral alkanizing agents to prevent hyperchloraemic acidosis.

There is an increase in the incidence of secondary malignancy at the site of uretero-colonic anastomosis. The risk is 22% at 20 years, and therefore these patients need regular surveillance of the reservoir after 12 years [23].

Continent urinary diversion – Mitrofanoff

This is the most demanding form of reconstructive surgery and there is a significant morbidity associated with this procedure. The Mitrofanoff principle refers to a system whereby a fine caliber tube, usually an appendix, acts as a catheterizable channel. One end is implanted via a submucosal tunnel into an orthotopic reconstructed bladder reservoir and the other is brought out to the surface as a cutaneous continent catheterizable stoma. Continence is achieved by bladder filling causing the tube to act as a flap valve, and the natural apposition of the mucosa of the Mitrofanoff tube.

The complication rate for this type of procedure is high, and 25% of patients will develop stenosis of the Mitrofanoff tube. Since the reservoir does not drain in a dependent manner, 10% of patients will develop reservoir calculi. Ninety percent will be continent [24].

Future developments

Laparoscopy has had a major impact upon the management of urological cancers, with the default technique for nephrectomy and prostatectomy now being laparoscopic. Cystectomy will almost certainly follow once the surgical skills are available.

Tissue engineering techniques have been used in benign disease to construct scaffolds for reconstruction with omental wraps to perform cystoplasties [25]. It is only a matter of time before the technical problems associated with using this technique in patients with malignant disease are overcome and these scaffolds are available for the construction of neobladders.

Conclusion

The surgical management of bladder cancer is dependent upon the stage and grade of the disease. Patients with superficial disease (except CIS) are managed with surveillance and endoscopic resection, whereas those with muscle invasive disease or persistent CIS need radical surgery. The surgical morbidity associated with cystectomy is significant; however, with improved surgical techniques it is hoped that patients will be able to achieve good long-term results both in terms of functional outcomes and cancer cure.

REFERENCES

1. Stein J P, Lieskovsky G, Cote R *et al.* Radical cystectomy in the treatment of invasive bladder cancer: long-term results in 1,054 patients. *J Clin Oncol* 2001; **19**: 666–75.
2. Pagano F, Bassi P, Galetti T P *et al.* Results of contemporary radical cystectomy for invasive bladder cancer: a clinicopathological study with an emphasis on the inadequacy of the tumor, nodes and metastases classification. *J Urol* 1991; **145**: 45–50.
3. Ghoneim M A, el-Mekresh M M, el-Baz M A *et al.* Radical cystectomy for carcinoma of the bladder: critical evaluation of the results in 1,026 cases. *J Urol* 1997; **158**: 393–9.
4. Lunacek A, Schwentner C, Fritsch H *et al.* Anatomical radical retropubic prostatectomy: "curtain dissection" of the neurovascular bundle. *BJU Int* 2005; **95**: 1226–31.
5. Marshall F F, Mostwin J L, Radebaugh L C *et al.* Ileocolic neobladder post-cystectomy: continence and potency. *J Urol* 1991; **145**: 502–4.
6. Schlegel P N, Walsh P C. Neuroanatomical approach to radical cystoprostatectomy with preservation of sexual function. *J Urol* 1987; **138**: 1402–6.
7. Chang S S, Cole E, Cookson M S *et al.* Preservation of the anterior vaginal wall during female radical cystectomy with orthotopic urinary diversion: technique and results. *J Urol* 2002; **168**: 1442–5.
8. Bhatta Dhar N, Kessler T M, Mills R D, Burkhard F, Studer U E. Nerve-sparing radical cystectomy and orthotopic bladder replacement in female patients. *Eur Urol* 2007 October; **52** (4): 1006–14. Epub March 5, 2007.

9. Mills R D, Studer U E. Female orthotopic bladder substitution: a good operation in the right circumstances. *J Urol* 2000; **163**: 1501–4.

10. Bhatt A, Nandipati K, Dhar N *et al.* Neurovascular preservation in orthotopic cystectomy: impact on female sexual function. *Urology* 2006; **67**: 742–5.

11. Nieuwenhuijzen J A, Meinhardt W, Horenblas S. Clinical outcomes after sexuality preserving cystectomy and neobladder (prostate sparing cystectomy) in 44 patients. *J Urol* 2005; **173**: 1314–17.

12. Vallancien G, Abou El Fettouh H, Cathelineau X *et al.* Cystectomy with prostate sparing for bladder cancer in 100 patients: 10-year experience. *J Urol* 2002; **168**: 2413–17.

13. Chahal R, Sundaram S K, Iddenden R *et al.* A study of the morbidity, mortality and long-term survival following radical cystectomy and radical radiotherapy in the treatment of invasive bladder cancer in Yorkshire. *Eur Urol* 2003; **43**: 246–57.

14. Nieuwenhuijzen J A, Horenblas S, Meinhardt W *et al.* Salvage cystectomy after failure of interstitial radiotherapy and external beam radiotherapy for bladder cancer. *BJU Int* 2004; **94**: 793–7.

15. Abol-Enein H, El-Baz M, AbdEl-Hameed M A *et al.* Lymph node involvement in patients with bladder cancer treated with radical cystectomy: a patho-anatomical study – a single center experience. *J Urol* 2004; **172**: 1818–21.

16. Abdel-Latif M, Abol-Enien H, El-Baz M, Ghoneim M A. Nodal involvement in bladder cancer cases treated with radical cystectomy: incidence and prognosis. *J Urol* 2004; **172**: 85–9.

17. Ghoneim M A, Abol-Enein H. Lymphadenectomy with cystectomy: is it necessary and what is its extent? *Eur Urol* 2004; **46**: 457–61.

18. Neal D E. Complications of ileal conduit diversion in adults with cancer followed up for at least five years. *Br Med J (Clin Res Ed)* 1985; **290**: 1695–7.

19. Madersbacher S, Schmidt J, Eberle J M *et al.* Long-term outcome of ileal conduit diversion. *J Urol* 2003; **169**: 985–90.

20. Perimenis P, Burkhard F C, Kessler T M *et al.* Ileal orthotopic bladder substitute combined with an afferent tubular segment: long-term upper urinary tract changes and voiding pattern. *Eur Urol* 2004; **46**: 604–9.

21. Hautmann R E, Volkmer B G, Schumacher M C *et al.* Long-term results of standard procedures in urology: the ileal neobladder. *World J Urol* 2006; **24**: 305–14.

22. Abol-Enein H, Ghoneim M A. Functional results of orthotopic ileal neobladder with serous-lined extramural ureteral reimplantation: experience with 450 patients. *J Urol* 2001; **165**: 1427–32.

23. D'elia G, Pahernik S, Fisch M *et al.* Mainz Pouch II technique: 10 years' experience. *BJU Int* 2004; **93**: 1037–42.

24. Wiesner C, Bonfig R, Stein R *et al.* Continent cutaneous urinary diversion: long-term follow-up of more than 800 patients with ileocecal reservoirs. *World J Urol* 2006: **24**: 315–18.

25. Atala A, Bauer S B, Soker S *et al.* Tissue-engineered autologous bladders for patients needing cystoplasty. *Lancet* 2006; **367**: 1241–6.

7

External beam radiotherapy for the treatment of muscle invasive bladder cancer

Susan Lalondrelle and Robert Huddart

Introduction

Options for the radical treatment of muscle invasive bladder cancer have traditionally been radical cystectomy or external beam radiotherapy. For many, cystectomy has been the preferred option, with radiotherapy given for medically inoperable cases [1]. Although no randomized comparison of the two treatments exists, outcomes with radiotherapy have historically been seen to be inferior [2–4]. This may have been owing to negative case selection, i.e. cases given radiotherapy being medically less fit or with poorer prognosis, and issues with stage migration in the comparison of clinically versus pathologically staged patients. More recent series, combining advances in systemic therapy and radiotherapy treatment planning and delivery, suggest comparable results to cystectomy [5–10] . The concept of selective bladder preservation is now gaining appeal, whereby radical treatment options are determined by the tumor response to neoadjuvant chemotherapy. As a result, more patients are undergoing radical radiotherapy and organ preservation.

Radiotherapy as a radical treatment for bladder cancer involves the delivery of a dose ("fraction") of high-energy X-rays (usually with peak voltage of 6–10 MV) to the target region of the bladder. This is repeated daily for four to six weeks to achieve a tumouricidal dose of radiation to the tumor itself while sparing surrounding normal tissue. The delivery of radiotherapy is technically demanding because of day-to-day variations in bladder filling, resulting in changes in bladder size and position, which must be accounted for to avoid geographic miss.

Carcinoma of the Bladder, ed. David MacVicar. Published by Cambridge University Press. © Cambridge University Press 2008.

Imaging techniques are central to success in this treatment at a number of key stages:

1. appropriate staging and disease delineation
2. target localization
3. verification of treatment delivery.

Delivery of radiotherapy is discussed in more detail in the sections that follow. Recent advances in radiotherapy treatment planning and delivery should help improve outcomes. Perhaps the greatest advance in the radiotherapy planning pathway over the last decade has been the introduction of three-dimensional CT planning for conformal delivery of radiation therapy, facilitating avoidance of irradiation of normal tissues and consequent escalation of dose to the primary tumor. By outlining target and normal tissues on consecutive CT slices, the radio-therapist can accurately define the regions to be treated and/or avoided by the radiation beams. This information is then analyzed and beam shaping designed (using lead blocks or, more commonly now, a device called a multileaf collimator) which maximizes normal tissue avoidance. Standard collimators use a solid lead jaw; a multileaf collimator uses a bank of lead "fingers" each 0.5–1 cm across and which can be moved independently. This allows irregular shaping of the field. Clinical trials have shown that this can reduce normal tissue toxicity compared to standard radiotherapy and can allow dose escalation. Advances in imaging should deliver further improvements by the way of allowing online imaging of internal organs between and during radiotherapy treatments ("image guidance"). Many organs, such as the bladder, are mobile structures and in the planning process safety margins are required to account for these uncertainties. Being more certain allows smaller margins to be used, less volume to be irradiated and (hopefully) lower toxicity and more effective treatments. A number of technologies are being investigated in this area but a key one is the development of reconstructed cross-sectional images (cone beam CT) using either the megavoltage treatment beam and/or a kilovoltage beam attached to the treatment machine.

Chemoradiotherapy

The observation that 40–60% of patients treated radically with cystectomy or radiotherapy relapse with systemic disease within 1–2 years [11] has prompted interest in chemotherapy strategies in bladder cancer treatment. Neoadjuvant chemotherapy results in pathological complete response rates of 48–75%, pre-dicting improved outcome with radiotherapy [8,12]. This observation and the radiosensitization effect seen with chemotherapy in other tumor sites have led to several phase II studies of concomitant radiotherapy and chemotherapy for bladder cancer. Using mostly cisplatin alone or in combination with 5FU, these have demonstrated the feasibility of such an approach without significant escalation of toxicity and improved outcomes compared to radiotherapy alone [9,13,14]. The only randomized trial has been conducted by the National Cancer Institute of Canada [15]. Ninety-nine patients were randomized between cisplatin and radiotherapy and radiotherapy alone to a dose of 40 Gy, followed by elective cystectomy or further radiotherapy. A non-significant improvement in complete response rate and overall survival was seen in the chemoradiotherapy arm. Pelvic recurrence was significantly reduced in the combined arm. Owing to concerns regarding the use of potentially nephrotoxic cisplatin in bladder cancer, the current UK National Cancer Research Network trial of concomitant chemoradiotherapy randomizes to radiotherapy alone or radiotherapy with mitomycin C and 5FU [16]. As bladder preservation strategies develop, it is likely that chemoradiotherapy will form an integral part of the trimodality approach to radical treatment (see Chapter 8).

The radiotherapy treatment planning pathway

Treating the patient with radiotherapy involves a number of clearly defined steps, which are described in the following sections.

Patient selection

Analyses of institutional series of radical radiotherapy to the bladder have highlighted several factors associated with improvement in outcome. These include disease-related factors such as earlier stage, lower grade, and the absence of pelvic nodal involvement; and patient factors such as younger age, normal renal function, absence of hydronephrosis and normal hemoglobin [3,17,18]. The most powerful positive predictive factor is maximal transurethral resection of bladder tumor (TURBT) [19] and thus as much tumor as safely possible should be resected at initial diagnosis.

Accurate staging of disease is vital in the selection of patients most likely to benefit from a bladder-preserving approach. In addition to cystoscopy, tumor staging investigations routinely include cross-sectional imaging with CT or MRI. Both techniques provide similar accuracy for tumor and nodal staging, although the higher contrast resolution with MRI may be better for smaller tumors [20].

Compared to clinical staging, MRI upstages muscle invasive disease in 30% of patients, which is correlated with worse outcomes following radiotherapy [21]. PET-CT provides a higher sensitivity for detecting distant metastases and increases the positive predictive factor for diagnosis of regional lymph node metastases compared to CT alone [22], but it is neither universally available nor accessible. SPECT-CT has been reported as a technique for the identification of sentinel nodes [23].

Defining the clinical target volume (CTV)

Once the patient has been selected for radiotherapy treatment, the radiotherapist must define the organs and structures to include as radiotherapy targets. Often, when planning radiotherapy, a gross tumor volume (GTV) is initially defined to represent the area of visible tumor which may then be expanded to include other structures and areas at risk of subclinical disease, termed the "clinical target volume," or CTV. The GTV is generally defined by a combination of cystoscopic assessment and imaging results (CT or MRI). For bladder tumors, the difficulty in distinguishing between tumor and post-resection inflammation limits the value of imaging for target definition. Thus, in the case of bladder cancer, where the GTV is not always clearly seen, it is common to delineate only the CTV. Whether newer techniques such as virtual cystoscopy could aid this delineation is unknown, and is subject to a current research project at our institution.

The key issues for the radiotherapist to decide are
1. whether or not to irradiate the pelvis to eradicate possible micrometastatic nodal disease,
2. whether to treat the entire mucosal surface of the bladder or just the tumor-bearing region, or a combination of both.

A two-phase technique, treating the pelvic lymph nodes, bladder, and proximal urethra to a lower dose and then boosting the tumor, results in large irradiated volumes, which will include small bowel and rectum. This may result in additional gastrointestinal toxicity. The more commonly utilized approach of treating the whole bladder (Figs. 7.1–7.3) and known extravesical disease in a single phase has never been compared in a randomized setting, but is not associated with inferior rates of local control [24]. Indeed, the use of neoadjuvant and/or concomitant chemotherapy may be sufficient to eradicate nodal disease while confining radiotherapy to the bladder itself.

Traditionally, the whole bladder has been included as target; however, the concept of partial bladder radiotherapy is currently gaining attention. This is based on the

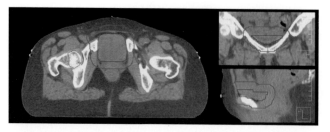

Figure 7.1 Axial, coronal and sagittal views of CT planning scan with clinical target volume (CTV) (blue) and planning target volume (PTV) (magenta) contoured (see also color plate section).

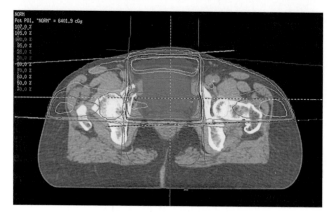

Figure 7.2 The margins of the three fields are outlined by red lines (AP field) at green and blue lines (lateral field). The planning target volume (PTV), shaded magenta, is placed over the area to be treated. Within this area the dose should be 95–105% of the dose at the isocenter of the volume. Each colored line represents an area of dose expressed as a percentage of the dose at the isocenter of PTV. These dose estimations are calculated from data acquired from phantom studies (see also color plate section).

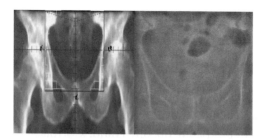

Figure 7.3 Digitally reconstructed radiograph of anterior treatment field and anterior portal image used for comparison of bony anatomy and verification of patient position.

observation that less than 8% of local relapse occurs at a new site within the bladder [25,26]. In addition, the tolerance of irradiated bladder mucosa is volume dependent – up to two-thirds of the bladder can receive 80 Gy, compared to 65 Gy if the whole organ is treated [27]. By reducing the volume of bladder and normal tissue receiving a high dose, acute and late toxicity will be limited [28], facilitating dose escalation to the tumor bed. Alternatively, a combination of these two approaches, treating the whole bladder followed by a boost to the tumor, is possible [29–31].

Tumor localization

After defining which areas are to be targeted, the next step in the production of the radiotherapy treatment plan is the localization and outlining of the target region (CTV) by the clinician. Conventional X-ray-based simulation using cystograms may result in geographic miss in up to 85% of cases [32] and has been superceded by CT-based planning. A CT scan of the pelvis with the patient in the treatment position is performed. An empty bladder is generally specified for whole bladder treatments as this results in reduced volumes and should be more reproducible on a day-to-day basis. The images are then transferred to the planning computer, where the clinician will outline the CTV. Where the CTV is the whole bladder, this is easily visualized on CT images (Fig. 7.1). The transition between bladder and prostate is less well visualized, resulting in some limited interobserver variability in delineation [33]. Delineation volumes also vary considerably between diagnostic radiologists and oncologists, with the former assigning a smaller CTV [34].

In order to localize a tumor boost, further information should be available in the form of surgical bladder maps, as following a maximal TURBT, bladder wall thickening may not be visible on cross-sectional imaging. As a radiotherapy planning tool, MRI has no proven benefit over CT. Ultrasound tomograms have also been used to accurately delineate tumor but would not constitute standard practice [35]. The use of intravenous contrast may enhance tumor localization, and a small volume of intravesicular contrast may also be used.

Organ motion and treatment margins

Daily variation is seen in the volume and position of the bladder and in the positioning of the patient so a further safety margin is added to the CTV to allow for this organ motion and set-up error. A number of studies have attempted to define the most appropriate margins to use based on observations of bladder motion using repeat CT scanning during radical treatment. The external influence of rectal volume results in a shift of bladder position, while bladder filling leads to shape changes [36]. This movement is seen predominantly in a superior and anterior direction with reported maximum excursions ranging from 5 to 36 mm [33,37–39]. Organ motion of this extent results in 10–42% of treatments being delivered off target [38,40,41] when standard 1.5–2 cm margins are used. Fokdal et al. [42] catheterized the rectum and bladder to study the effects of bladder motion. With a large rectal volume and full bladder, a margin of 3.5 cm was required in the caudal direction. Others have attempted to use "margin recipes" to define anisotropic margins [38] but motion is also dependent on the tumor position and size [40,43], thus assuming generic margins is hazardous.

Intrafraction motion, i.e. displacement, over time from bladder emptying to the end of treatment delivery is not generally included in margin calculations but can be significant. Depending on individual urinary inflow rates, bladder volume may increase up to 90 cc in 10 minutes, causing a 2 cm shift [39,44,45].

Set-up error describes the variation in patient position, which may be either random or systematic. Few studies have addressed this issue in bladder cancer. Using electronic portal images (EPI) bony anatomy can be aligned to simulator films or digitally reconstructed radiographs generated from planning CT scans. On average, errors >0.5 cm occur in 24–33% of treatments imaged in a superior–inferior direction and in 15–21% in a right to left direction [46,47]. Additional margins of 2–6 mm are thought sufficient to account for set-up error [33,38].

There is no doubt that there is marked individual variation of bladder motion, determined by post-micturition volumes, urinary inflow rates, rectal volumes and tumor size and position. Current standard margins of 2 cm are insufficient in some cases and unnecessarily generous in others. The future goals of radiotherapy in bladder cancer must be to optimize treatment margins on an individual basis based on the above factors and to ensure better day-to-day positioning. This will not only ensure that 100% of treatments are delivered on target, but will limit normal tissue exposure and allow dose escalation to be investigated.

Conformal radiotherapy and intensity-modulated radiotherapy for the bladder

Having defined a planning target volume (PTV) of tissue to be irradiated, the goal of the physicist is to produce a treatment plan that delivers the prescribed dose precisely to that volume. Conformal radiotherapy refers to the ability to shape the dose around the 3-D target, resulting in reduced normal tissue toxicity and facilitating dose escalation [48]. This has become a reality in the last decade with the advent of computerized planning systems and multileaf collimation (MLC) based on CT scan data. Multileaf collimation uses 0.5–1 cm individual "fingers" of lead to collimate the beam, allowing irregularly shaped beam delivery. Computerized planning systems allow the planner to design treatment portals based on the corresponding volume surface and to view the resultant dose homogeneity across the entire target. Treatment delivery and the manipulation of MLC leaves are directly under the guidance of the same computer, avoiding the potential for manual error in manufacture and use of shaped lead blocks. A typical bladder plan uses a three (one anterior and two lateral or posterior obliques) (Fig. 7.2) or four (anterior, posterior and two opposed laterals) field beam arrangement to deliver dose to the pelvis.

Intensity-modulated radiotherapy (IMRT) delivers the ultimate conformal treatment. Standard radiotherapy uses a uniform dose flux across the treatment portal but in IMRT the dose intensity can be varied across each field. Multiple beams are employed in order to improve conformality and dose homogeneity across the target volume. IMRT is most commonly planned using an inverse-planning rather than a conventional forward-planning technique. In forward planning, an approximation is made of the treatment fields based on experience and training, with modifications to optimize the planned dose to the target volume. In inverse planning, the treatment goals in terms of the dose distribution and normal tissue toxicity dose limits are assigned with computerized optimization of beam arrangements and intensity patterns. IMRT has been proven feasible in bladder cancer [49], and when planned as a boost volume it may reduce the volume of normal tissue irradiated by high dose by 76%, which is achievable with a five or seven beam arrangement [31]. An increased number of beams should result in a larger volume of normal tissue receiving lower dose radiation, although this has unknown long-term consequences.

Dose and fractionation

Once the volume to be treated is determined, the dose/fractionation schedule to be used has to be decided. Variables to consider when choosing a regime are the total biologically effective dose, overall time, treatment volume and the concomitant use of chemotherapy. The most commonly employed regimes are 60–66 Gy in 2 Gy fractions over six to six and a half weeks or 52.5–55 Gy in 20 fractions over four weeks. A total biologically effective dose below 60 Gy is associated with poorer outcomes, and a dose–response relationship has been observed clinically for transitional cell carcinoma [50,51]. Radiobiological modeling suggests that an incremental increase of 1 Gy above 60 Gy is associated with an improvement in local control of 6% and in overall survival of 7.5% at five years [52]. Using data derived from published studies of external beam radiotherapy, Pos *et al.* [53] have estimated a 10% improvement in local control, from 50 to 60%, for an increase in total dose by 10 Gy. Attempts to achieve dose escalation using standard fractionation clinically have, however, been hampered by the coincident increase in normal tissue toxicity.

Prolongation of treatment time is associated with inferior outcomes in other tumor sites but conflicting evidence exists in the case of bladder cancer [52–54]. A number of methods have been tested to try to improve therapeutic gain. Reducing the overall time, termed "acceleration," theoretically reduces tumor repopulation, resulting in less cancer to kill and better results. Acceleration is achieved by increasing the number of fractions (hyperfractionation) or increasing the dose per fraction (hypofractionation). Hyperfractionation and acceleration have failed to show significant improvements in outcome, and result in increased acute gastrointestinal toxicity [30,55,56]. Hypofractionation may increase late toxicity [57]. A further way to escalate the dose to the tumor and reduce overall time is through a concomitant boost. The first fraction of therapy is delivered to the whole pelvis, followed more than six hours later by a further fraction to the whole bladder or tumor. Feasibility of such an approach has been demonstrated, also in combination with chemotherapy [29,30,58,59], with complete response rates of 74–80% and three-year survival of 46–61%. This does not appear to result in additional acute or late toxicity.

Treatment delivery and verification

Following production of an appropriate treatment plan, radiotherapy is delivered to the patient. As for treatment planning, radiotherapy is delivered in the supine position, without immobilization, to an empty bladder. Skin tattoos serve to align the patient in the same position each time. Standard practice consists of electronic portal images being acquired on the first three to five days of treatment and then weekly depending on departmental guidelines. These megavoltage (MV) images, which can be acquired during treatment delivery or as an additional dose, provide a radiographic documentation of bony anatomy position. They are correlated with digitally reconstructed radiographs from the CT planning scan to ascertain systematic and random set-up errors (Fig. 7.3). This review process is usually performed offline, or retrospectively, with systematic error corrected using a couch shift prior to subsequent treatments. This process does not provide any information relating to the position of the pelvic organs themselves.

An empty bladder should be reproducible on a daily basis but time delays and incomplete voiding of diseased bladders result in varying degrees of bladder filling and thus potential displacement of the target out of the treatment field. Current research is focused on this issue and on addressing whether the use of soft tissue imaging during the course of radiotherapy can improve the quality of treatment.

Three-dimensional CT images can be obtained either immediately before or after treatment delivery to document the position of the target and organs at risk and to assess changes to patient and tumor anatomy as a consequence of treatment. This is achievable with a variety of applications available with new generation linear accelerators. The Siemens Primatom is an example of a "CT on rails", i.e. a diagnostic-quality CT scanner matched to the axis of the linear accelerator using the flat bed of the treatment table. This has the advantage of superior image quality but requires much more space than a standard linear accelerator. The tomotherapy unit has the appearance of a diagnostic scanner gantry and the linear accelerator component is adapted to deliver helical IMRT [60]. Combined with adaptive software, automated correction of patient position is possible. The image quality from the megavoltage X-ray beam is, however, inferior to conventional CT and image acquisition times can be lengthy.

    The most widely utilized solution is cone beam CT, whereby the X-ray source is integrated into the linear accelerator gantry either within the head or at 90° and the 2-D flat-panel X-ray detector lies opposite. In a 180° or 360° rotation of the gantry around the patient, hundreds of projections are acquired to image an area of up to 26 cm in superior–inferior extent in 1–2 minutes (Fig. 7.4). Both kilovoltage and megavoltage sources are commercially available, with kilovoltage providing marginally better image quality but at the expense of additional dose [61]. One gantry rotation of cone beam CT generates a dataset of a larger volume in comparison to fan beam CT, which generates a dataset for one slice with each rotation. The volumetric reconstruction of the projections is performed as a parallel process using a modified Feldkamp algorithm. Image quality from cone beam CT is not yet comparable to diagnostic imaging owing to X-ray scatter effect generating artifact, although several solutions to this problem are being investigated [62]. The immediate application of these systems is in online evaluation of patient alignment. Cone beam images can be matched to the planning CT scan either in bone or soft tissue windows and set-up errors corrected prior to delivery of each fraction. The utility of cone beam imaging

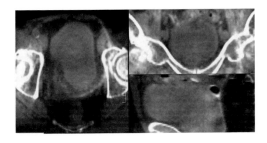

Figure 7.4 Axial, coronal and sagittal views of reconstructed cone beam images.

in verification of bony and soft tissue position has been established for most tumor sites [63]. This process adds a further 8–10 mins. to the daily treatment time and for this reason is not feasible on such a frequent basis.

Image-guided adaptive planning

The commercial availability of cone beam applications is a significant step toward a solution to the problem of organ and tumor position variability during a radical course of treatment. Serial imaging with cone beam CT allows a patient-specific profile of organ motion to be established, which can then be used to assign more appropriate margins to the CTV. During therapy, the tumor may also be seen to regress, resulting in changes to patient contours and irradiation of normal tissue unnecessarily. Various methods of adapting the treatment fields during the course of therapy have now been described. Although most work is described in relation to prostate cancer, the bladder provides an ideal model for adaptive radiotherapy as individual plans can be generated based on patterns of bladder filling and deformity. Using serial CT images to evaluate the maximal excursions of the prostate gland over the first five days of treatment, Yan *et al.* [64] described the first offline adaptive process. By creating a volume that encompassed all the possible positions of the gland, the large internal organ motion margin that is generically added to the CTV was removed and the only further margin added was to account for set-up error. The new "adapted" plan is implemented during the second week of treatment and its accuracy ensured through weekly repeat scans. Consequently, reductions in PTV of up to 40% were seen, facilitating dose escalation without an increase in chronic rectal toxicity [65,66]. This method has also been reported by Nuver *et al.* [67] from the Netherlands, who found a reduction in PTV volume of on average 30% and required margins of 7 mm around the CTV. The same group have investigated an adaptive process for partial bladder radiotherapy and demonstrated the feasibility of this leading to reduction in PTV volumes of 40% [68]. This impressive reduction in the PTV can only be achieved with additional time for the acquisition of imaging and physics recalculation and has yet to be translated into a clinical endpoint. An alternative and online method is to predict the individual's bladder filling pattern through cine-MRI or serial CT and design a series of radiotherapy treatment plans based on this. Following acquisition of cone beam imaging pre-treatment, the most appropriate plan can be selected for that day and implemented. This has in part been reported in using differential margins added to the planning scan CTV [69], with plan selection based on cone beam imaging days 1–5 and weekly. This plan selection method resulted in a $31\,cm^3$ reduction (SD $+/-23\,cm^3$) in the PTV on average. Future developments will focus on a fully automated method of cone beam fusion, assessment and adaptation of treatment plans on a daily basis [70,71]. This will permit each fraction of radiotherapy to be delivered to the target with greater certainty, paving the way for clinical trials of dose escalation.

Toxicity

Side effects from radical radiotherapy to the urinary bladder are classified as acute (occurring during and shortly after treatment completion) and late (occurring months to years following completion of treatment). A grading of severity is assigned according to the Radiotherapy and Oncology Group (RTOG) scoring systems (Table 7.1).

Acute urinary complications in the form of dysuria, hematuria and frequency are common, occurring in around 20% of patients [72], although hematuria related to persistent tumor will often resolve. Diarrhea occurs in up to 30%, often requiring treatment. Fatigue may be limited by ensuring adequate hemoglobin concentration throughout treatment.

Both urinary and gastrointestinal late side effects may occur. The most-recent, large, single institution series published of 459 patients treated with radical radiotherapy found the incidence of late gastrointestinal and urinary side effects to be 6.1 and 23% respectively [72]. These are predominantly grade 1 and 2, with only 0.4% incidence of late gastrointestinal side effect in the form of rectal bleeding and intestinal obstruction. Urinary grade 3 and 4 toxicity is also rare (2.6 and 0.6% respectively), and occurs in the form of severe dysuria, hematuria and chronic ulcero-necrotic cystitis. The use of dose-volume histograms aids the clinician's evaluation of the treatment plan in terms of the likelihood of toxicity. Acceptable limits are defined by a 5% incidence of severe late effects at five years according to work by Emami *et al.* [27]. However, motion of the organs at risk as well as the target reduces the reliability of this method, as rectal and bladder volumes are based on the snapshot image of the planning CT scan. Again, further knowledge of organ position at the time of radiotherapy delivery is vital for accurate modelling of toxicity and outcomes.

Palliative radiotherapy

In the setting of metastatic disease or medical comorbidity where the aim of local treatment is relief of symptoms, radiotherapy can also be beneficial. Short courses

Table 7.1. Radiotherapy and Oncology Group scoring system for acute and late radiation toxicity

	RTOG score					
	Grade 0	Grade 1	Grade 2	Grade 3	Grade 4	Grade 5
Acute genito-urinary	No change	Frequency of urination or nocturia twice pre-treatment habit/dysuria, urgency not requiring medication	Frequency of urination or nocturia which is less frequent than every hour. Dysuria, urgency, bladder spasm requiring local anesthetic (e.g. Pyridium)	Frequency with urgency and nocturia hourly or more frequently/dysuria, pelvis pain or bladder spasm requiring regular, frequent narcotic/gross hematuria with/without clot passage	Hematuria requiring transfusion/ acute bladder obstruction not secondary to clot passage, ulceration or necrosis	Death directly related to radiation late effects
Acute gastro-intestinal	No change	Increased frequency or change in quality of bowel habits not requiring medication/rectal discomfort not requiring analgesics	Diarrhea requiring parasympatholytic drugs (e.g. Lomotil)/mucous discharge not necessitating sanitary pads/rectal or abdominal pain requiring analgesics	Diarrhea requiring parenteral support/severe mucous or blood discharge necessitating sanitary pads/abdominal distension (flat plate radiograph demonstrates distended bowel loops)	Acute or subacute obstruction, fistula or perforation; GI bleeding requiring transfusion; abdominal pain or tenesmus requiring tube decompression or bowel diversion	
Late bladder	None	Slight epithelial atrophy. Minor telangiectasia (microscopic hematuria)	Moderate frequency. Generalized telangiectasia, intermittent macroscopic hematuria	Severe frequency and dysuria. Severe generalized telangiectasia (often with petechiae). Frequent hematuria and reduction in bladder capacity (<150 cc)	Necrosis/contracted bladder (capacity < 100 cc). Severe hemorrhagic cystitis	
Late bowel	None	Mild diarrhea, mild cramping, bowel movement five times daily, slight rectal discharge or bleeding	Moderate diarrhea and colic, bowel movement > 5 times daily, excessive rectal mucus or intermittent bleeding	Obstruction or bleeding requiring surgery	Necrosis/perforation, fistula	

of hypofractionated treatment are used to avoid the burden of daily attendance. Although hypofractionated treatment may result in increased late toxicity, this is balanced by the poor prognosis of such patients. Symptoms of hematuria, frequency and pain may all be relieved with a variety of fractionations: 30–36 Gy in five or six weekly fractions, 17–21 Gy in two or three weekly fractions or 30 Gy in ten daily fractions all achieve palliation of hematuria in 52–85% of patients and palliation of local pain in 52–68% [73–75]. The target volume is usually the whole bladder and any obvious extravesical extension with a standard 1.5 to 2 cm margin. Data on acute toxicity associated with palliative regimes is sparse. The incidence of late toxicity has been observed to be 7–9% [74,76]. However, studies that have reported these levels include patients with T1 and T2 disease without symptoms, representing a better prognosis group with longer follow-up.

External beam radiotherapy is also of use in the palliation of painful bone metastases from primary bladder cancer.

Summary

External beam radiotherapy is an established organ-preserving treatment option in the radical management of bladder cancer. Outcomes may improve with the use of neoadjuvant chemotherapy to determine the most suitable patients for this approach and of concurrent chemotherapy for radiosensitization. Advances in radiotherapy planning and delivery will deliver more precise treatment. The introduction of serial soft tissue imaging during the course of radical treatment will demonstrate individual bladder filling patterns and target variation, ensuring that treatment is given on target. Adapting radiotherapy fields based on these observations will allow dose escalation to be investigated, with the possibility of improved local control and survival. There are many steps in the radiotherapy pathway where accurate imaging is key and close collaboration between oncology and radiology will aid further progress.

REFERENCES

1. Bales G T, Kim H, Steinberg G D. Surgical therapy for locally advanced bladder cancer. *Semin Oncol* 1996; **23**: 605–13.
2. Shelley M D, Barber J, Wilt T, Mason M D. Surgery versus radiotherapy for muscle invasive bladder cancer. *Cochrane Database Syst Rev* 2002; **1**: CD002079.

3. Gospodarowicz M K, Hawkins N V, Rawlings G A *et al.* Radical radiotherapy for muscle invasive transitional cell carcinoma of the bladder: failure analysis. *J Urol* 1989; **142**: 1448–53; discussion 1453–4.

4. Duncan W, Quilty P M. The results of a series of 963 patients with transitional cell carcinoma of the urinary bladder primarily treated by radical megavoltage X-ray therapy. *Radiother Oncol* 1986; **7**: 299–310.

5. Dunst J, Diestelhorst A, Kuhn R *et al.* Organ-sparing treatment in muscle-invasive bladder cancer. *Strahlenther Onkol* 2005; **181**: 632–7.

6. Rodel C, Grabenbauer G G, Kuhn R *et al.* Organ preservation in patients with invasive bladder cancer: initial results of an intensified protocol of transurethral surgery and radiation therapy plus concurrent cisplatin and 5-fluorouracil. *Int J Radiat Oncol Biol Phys* 2002; **52**: 1303–9.

7. Shipley W U, Kaufman D S, Zehr E *et al.* Selective bladder preservation by combined modality protocol treatment: long-term outcomes of 190 patients with invasive bladder cancer. *Urology* 2002; **60**: 62–7; discussion 67–8.

8. Shipley W U, Winter K A, Kaufman D S *et al.* Phase III trial of neoadjuvant chemotherapy in patients with invasive bladder cancer treated with selective bladder preservation by combined radiation therapy and chemotherapy: initial results of Radiation Therapy Oncology Group 89–03. *J Clin Oncol* 1998; **16**: 3576–83.

9. Tester W, Porter A, Asbell S *et al.* Combined modality program with possible organ preservation for invasive bladder carcinoma: results of RTOG protocol 85–12. *Int J Radiat Oncol Biol Phys* 1993; **25**: 783–90.

10. Housset M, Maulard C, Chretien Y *et al.* Combined radiation and chemotherapy for invasive transitional-cell carcinoma of the bladder: a prospective study. *J Clin Oncol* 1993; **11**: 2150–7.

11. Prout G R Jr., Griffin P P, Shipley W U. Bladder carcinoma as a systemic disease. *Cancer* 1979; **43**: 2532–9.

12. Sternberg C N, Pansadoro V, Calabro F *et al.* Can patient selection for bladder preservation be based on response to chemotherapy? *Cancer* 2003; **97**: 1644–52.

13. Housset M, Dufour B, Durdux C *et al.* Concurrent radio-chemotherapy in infiltrating cancer of the bladder: a new therapeutic approach? *Cancer Radiother* 1998; **2**(suppl 1): 67s–72s.

14. Chauvet B, Felix-Faure C, Davin J L *et al.* Results of long-term treatment of inoperable cancer of the bladder with cisplatin and concurrent irradiation: prognostic factors of local control and survival. *Cancer Radiother* 1998; **2**(suppl 1): 85s–91s.

15. Coppin C, Gospodarowicz M. The NCI-Canada trial of concurrent cisplatin and radiotherapy for muscle invasive bladder cancer. *Prog Clin Biol Res* 1990; **353**: 75–83.

16. A randomised phase III study of radiotherapy with and without synchronous chemotherapy in muscle invasive bladder cancer – BC2001, www.bc2001.org.uk

17. Shipley W U, Rose M A. Bladder cancer. The selection of patients for treatment by full-dose irradiation. *Cancer* 1985; **55**(9 suppl): 2278–84.

18. Quilty P M, Kerr G R, Duncan W. Prognostic indices for bladder cancer: an analysis of patients with transitional cell carcinoma of the bladder primarily treated by radical megavoltage X-ray therapy. *Radiother Oncol* 1986; **7**: 311–21.

19. Rodel C, Grabenbauer G G, Kuhn R *et al*. Combined-modality treatment and selective organ preservation in invasive bladder cancer: long-term results. *J Clin Oncol* 2002; **20**: 3061–71.

20. MacVicar A D. Bladder cancer staging. *BJU Int* 2000; **86**(suppl 1): 111–22.

21. Robinson P, Collins C D, Ryder W D *et al*. Relationship of MRI and clinical staging to outcome in invasive bladder cancer treated by radiotherapy. *Clin Radiol* 2000; **55**: 301–6.

22. Drieskens O, Oyen R, van Poppel H *et al*. FDG-PET for preoperative staging of bladder cancer. *Eur J Nucl Med Mol Imaging* 2005; **32**: 1412–17.

23. Sherif A, Garske U, de la Torre M, Thorne M. Hybrid SPECT-CT: an additional technique for sentinel node detection of patients with invasive bladder cancer. *Eur Urol* 2006; **50**: 83–91.

24. Sengelov L, von der Maase H. Radiotherapy in bladder cancer. *Radiother Oncol* 1999; **52**: 1–14.

25. Cowan R A, McBain C A, Ryder W D *et al*. Radiotherapy for muscle-invasive carcinoma of the bladder: results of a randomized trial comparing conventional whole bladder with dose-escalated partial bladder radiotherapy. *Int J Radiat Oncol Biol Phys* 2004; **59**: 197–207.

26. van der Werf-Messing B, Menon R S, Hop W C. Carcinoma of the urinary bladder category T3NxMo treated by the combination of radium implant and external irradiation: second report. *Int J Radiat Oncol Biol Phys* 1983; **9**: 177–80.

27. Emami B, Lyman J, Brown A *et al*. Tolerance of normal tissue to therapeutic irradiation. *Int J Radiat Oncol Biol Phys* 1991; **21**: 109–22.

28. Mangar S A, Foo K, Norman A *et al*. Evaluating the effect of reducing the high-dose volume on the toxicity of radiotherapy in the treatment of bladder cancer. *Clin Oncol (R Coll Radiol)* 2006; **18**: 466–73.

29. Pos F J, van Tienhoven G, Hulshof M C *et al*. Concomitant boost radiotherapy for muscle invasive bladder cancer. *Radiother Oncol* 2003; **68**: 75–80.

30. Yavuz A A, Uavuz M N, Ozgur G K *et al*. Accelerated superfractionated radiotherapy with concomitant boost for invasive bladder cancer. *Int J Radiat Oncol Biol Phys* 2003; **56**: 734–45.

31. Muren L P, Redpath A T, McLaren D *et al*. A concomitant tumour boost in bladder irradiation: patient suitability and the potential of intensity-modulated radiotherapy. *Radiother Oncol* 2006; **80**: 98–105.

32. Rothwell R I, Ash D V, Jones W G. Radiation treatment planning for bladder cancer: a comparison of cystogram localisation with computed tomography. *Clin Radiol* 1983; **34**: 103–11.

33. Meijer G J, Rasch C, Remeijer P, Lebesque J V. Three-dimensional analysis of delineation errors, setup errors, and organ motion during radiotherapy of bladder cancer. *Int J Radiat Oncol Biol Phys* 2003; **55**: 1277–87.

34. Logue J P, Sharrock C L, Cowan R A *et al*. Clinical variability of target volume description in conformal radiotherapy planning. *Int J Radiat Oncol Biol Phys* 1998; **41**: 929–31.

35. Perkins A C, Price H M, Cox D J et al. Ultrasound in the localisation of bladder tumours for radiotherapy treatment planning. *Br J Radiol* 1984; **57**: 241–5.

36. Lotz H T, Remeijer P, van Herk M et al. A model to predict bladder shapes from changes in bladder and rectal filling. *Med Phys* 2004; **31**: 1415–23.

37. Turner S L, Swindell R, Bowl N et al. Bladder movement during radiation therapy for bladder cancer: implications for treatment planning. *Int J Radiat Oncol Biol Phys* 1997; **39**: 355–60.

38. Muren L P, Smaaland R, Dahl O. Organ motion, set-up variation and treatment margins in radical radiotherapy of urinary bladder cancer. *Radiother Oncol* 2003; **69**: 291–304.

39. Lotz H T, van Herk M, Betgen A et al. Reproducibility of the bladder shape and bladder shape changes during filling. *Med Phys* 2005; **32**: 2590–7.

40. Pos F J, Koedooder K, Hulshof M C et al. Influence of bladder and rectal volume on spatial variability of a bladder tumor during radical radiotherapy. *Int J Radiat Oncol Biol Phys* 2003; **55**: 835–41.

41. Sur R K, Clinkard J, Jones W G et al. Changes in target volume during radiotherapy treatment of invasive bladder carcinoma. *Clin Oncol (R Coll Radiol)* 1993; **5**: 30–3.

42. Fokdal L, Honore H, Hoyer M et al. Impact of changes in bladder and rectal filling volume on organ motion and dose distribution of the bladder in radiotherapy for urinary bladder cancer. *Int J Radiat Oncol Biol Phys* 2004; **59**: 436–44.

43. Lotz H T, Pos F J, Hulshof M C et al. Tumor motion and deformation during external radiotherapy of bladder cancer. *Int J Radiat Oncol Biol Phys* 2006; **64**: 1551–8.

44. McBain C A, Buckley D L, Amer A et al. Optimising bladder radiotherapy: MR assessment of time-dependant organ motion. *Clin Oncol* 2003; **15**(suppl 2): S13.

45. Mangar S, Huddart R, Sohaib A et al. Assessing intrafractional bladder motion using cine-MRI as initial methodology for Predictive Organ Localization (POLO) in radiotherapy for bladder cancer. *Radiother Oncol* 2007; **85**: 207–14.

46. Hanna C L, Slade S, Mason M D, Burnett N G. Accuracy of patient positioning during radiotherapy for bladder and brain tumours. *Clin Oncol (R Coll Radiol)* 1999; **11**: 93–8.

47. Huddart R A, Nahum A, Neal A et al. Accuracy of pelvic radiotherapy: prospective analysis of 90 patients in a randomised trial of blocked versus standard radiotherapy. *Radiother Oncol* 1996; **39**: 19–29.

48. Dearnaley D P, Khoo V S, Norman A R et al. Comparison of radiation side-effects of conformal and conventional radiotherapy in prostate cancer: a randomised trial. *Lancet* 1999; **353**: 267–72.

49. Budgell G J, Mott J H, Logue J P, Hounsell A R. Clinical implementation of dynamic multileaf collimation for compensated bladder treatments. *Radiother Oncol* 2001; **59**: 31–8.

50. Maciejewski B, Majewski S. Dose fractionation and tumour repopulation in radiotherapy for bladder cancer. *Radiother Oncol* 1991; **21**: 163–70.

51. Morrison R. The results of treatment of cancer of the bladder: a clinical contribution to radiobiology. *Clin Radiol* 1975; **26**: 67–75.

52. Majewski W, Maciejewski B, Majewski S et al. Clinical radiobiology of stage T2-T3 bladder cancer. *Int J Radiat Oncol Biol Phys* 2004; **60**: 60–70.

53. Pos F J, Hart G, Schneider C, Sminia P. Radical radiotherapy for invasive bladder cancer: what dose and fractionation schedule to choose? *Int J Radiat Oncol Biol Phys* 2006; **64**: 1168–73.

54. Moonen L, vd Voet H, de Nijs R et al. Muscle-invasive bladder cancer treated with external beam radiation: influence of total dose, overall treatment time, and treatment interruption on local control. *Int J Radiat Oncol Biol Phys* 1998; **42**: 525–30.

55. Horwich A, Dearnaley D, Huddart R et al. A randomized trial of accelerated radiotherapy for localised invasive bladder cancer. *Radiother Oncol* 2005; **75**: 34–43.

56. Moonen L, van der Voet H, Horenblas S, Bartelink H. A feasibility study of accelerated fractionation in radiotherapy of carcinoma of the urinary bladder. *Int J Radiat Oncol Biol Phys* 1997; **37**: 537–42.

57. Scholten A N, Leer J W, Collins C D et al. Hypofractionated radiotherapy for invasive bladder cancer. *Radiother Oncol* 1997; **43**: 163–9.

58. Hagan M P, Winter K A, Kaufman D S et al. RTOG 97–06: initial report of a phase I-II trial of selective bladder conservation using TURBT, twice-daily accelerated irradiation sensitized with cisplatin, and adjuvant MCV combination chemotherapy. *Int J Radiat Oncol Biol Phys* 2003; **57**: 665–72.

59. Zouhair A, Oszahin M, Schneider D et al. Invasive bladder carcinoma: a pilot study of conservative treatment with accelerated radiotherapy and concomitant cisplatin. *Int J Cancer* 2001; **96**: 350–5.

60. Ruchala K J, Olivera G H, Schloesser E A, Mackie T. Megavoltage CT on a tomotherapy system. *Phys Med Biol* 1999; **44**: 2597–621.

61. Jaffray D, Kupelian P, Djemil T, Macklis R M. Review of image-guided radiation therapy. *Expert Rev Anticancer Ther* 2007; **7**: 89–103.

62. Letourneau D, Wong R, Moseley D et al. Online planning and delivery technique for radiotherapy of spinal metastases using cone-beam CT: image quality and system performance. *Int J Radiat Oncol Biol Phys* 2007; **67**: 1229–37.

63. McBain C A, Henry A M, Sykes J et al. X-ray volumetric imaging in image-guided radiotherapy: the new standard in on-treatment imaging. *Int J Radiat Oncol Biol Phys* 2006; **64**: 625–34.

64. Yan D, Lockman D, Brabbins D et al. An off-line strategy for constructing a patient-specific planning target volume in adaptive treatment process for prostate cancer. *Int J Radiat Oncol Biol Phys* 2000; **48**: 289–302.

65. Brabbins D, Martinez A, Yan D et al. A dose-escalation trial with the adaptive radiotherapy process as a delivery system in localized prostate cancer: analysis of chronic toxicity. *Int J Radiat Oncol Biol Phys* 2005; **61**: 400–8.

66. Vargas C, Yan D, Kestin L L et al. Phase II dose escalation study of image-guided adaptive radiotherapy for prostate cancer: use of dose-volume constraints to achieve rectal isotoxicity. *Int J Radiat Oncol Biol Phys* 2005; **63**: 141–9.

67. Nuver T T, Hoogeman M S, Remeijer P *et al.* An adaptive off-line procedure for radiotherapy of prostate cancer. *Int J Radiat Oncol Biol Phys* 2007; **67**: 1559–67.

68. Pos F J, Hulshof M, Lebesque J *et al.* Adaptive radiotherapy for invasive bladder cancer: a feasibility study. *Int J Radiat Oncol Biol Phys* 2006; **64**: 862–8.

69. Burridge N, Amer A, Marchant T *et al.* Online adaptive radiotherapy of the bladder: small bowel irradiated-volume reduction. *Int J Radiat Oncol Biol Phys* 2006; **66**: 892–7.

70. Court L E, Tishler R B, Petit J *et al.* Automatic online adaptive radiation therapy techniques for targets with significant shape change: a feasibility study. *Phys Med Biol* 2006; **51**: 2493–501.

71. Court L E, Dong L, Lee A K *et al.* An automatic CT-guided adaptive radiation therapy technique by online modification of multileaf collimator leaf positions for prostate cancer. *Int J Radiat Oncol Biol Phys* 2005; **62**: 154–63.

72. Tonoli S, Bertoni F, De Stefani A *et al.* Radical radiotherapy for bladder cancer: retrospective analysis of a series of 459 patients treated in an Italian institution. *Clin Oncol (R Coll Radiol)* 2006; **18**: 52–9.

73. McLaren D B, Morrey D, Mason M D. Hypofractionated radiotherapy for muscle invasive bladder cancer in the elderly. *Radiother Oncol* 1997; **43**: 171–4.

74. Rostom A Y, Tahir S, Gershuny A R *et al.* Once weekly irradiation for carcinoma of the bladder. *Int J Radiat Oncol Biol Phys* 1996; **35**: 289–92.

75. Duchesne G M, Bolger J J, Griffiths G O *et al.* A randomized trial of hypofractionated schedules of palliative radiotherapy in the management of bladder carcinoma: results of medical research council trial BA09. *Int J Radiat Oncol Biol Phys* 2000; **47**: 379–88.

76. Holmang S, Borghede G. Early complications and survival following short-term palliative radiotherapy in invasive bladder carcinoma. *J Urol* 1996; **155**: 100–2.

8

The chemotherapeutic management of bladder cancer

Delia Pudney, Joanne Stokoe and Robert Huddart

Introduction

Approximately 20% of patients diagnosed with bladder cancer have muscle invasion at the time of presentation, and up to 50% of these patients will develop metastatic disease after successful local treatment. Bladder cancer is a relatively chemosensitive disease, with objective response rates of up to 25% with single agent chemotherapy and response rates of up to 50% with combination chemotherapy. The most commonly used regimens have historically been those combining cisplatin, methotrexate, vinca alkaloids and doxorubicin. In more recent years, the development of newer agents has led trials examining the role of gemcitabine and docetaxel as first- and second-line treatment for advanced bladder cancer. Care must be taken in delivering chemotherapy to patients with significant renal impairment as cisplatin is renally toxic, and methotrexate is excreted via the kidneys. In patients with renal insufficiency, carboplatin can be substituted for cisplatin and plasma methotrexate levels should be monitored and folinic acid rescue employed to prevent life-threatening toxicity.

Chemotherapy for bladder cancer is used in the neoadjuvant and adjuvant setting in combination with radical local treatment (cystectomy or radiotherapy) or for palliation in patients with advanced disease. Concurrent chemotherapy with radiotherapy has also been given with the aim of improving the therapeutic ratio of radical radiotherapy. Table 8.1 describes the scheduling of the chemotherapy regimens commonly used for the management of bladder cancer.

Neoadjuvant chemotherapy

Neoadjuvant chemotherapy has two potential therapeutic benefits: to improve the likelihood of bladder preservation and to eradicate micrometastatic disease. The

Table 8.1. Summary of the commonly used chemotherapy regimens in the management of bladder cancer

CMV	Methotrexate 40 mg/m^2 days 1 and 8 Vinblastine 5 mg/m^2 days 1 and 8 Cisplatin 100 mg/m^2 day 2 Cycle repeated every 21 days
M-VAC	Methotrexate 30 mg/m^2 days 2, 15 and 22 Vinblastine 3 mg/m^2 days 2, 15 and 22 Adriamycin 30 mg/m^2 day 2 Cisplatin 70 mg/m^2 day 2 Cycle repeated every 28 days
Accelerated M-VAC	Methotrexate 30 mg/m^2 day 1 Vinblastine 3 mg/m^2 day 2 Adriamycin 30 mg/m^2 day 2 Cisplatin 70 mg/m^2 day 2 Cycle repeated every 14 days G-CSF given d4–11 each cycle
Gemcitabine/cisplatin	Gemcitabine 1000 mg/m^2 days 1, 8 and 15 Cisplatin 70 mg/m^2 day 2 Cycle repeated every 28 days

five-year survival following radical cystectomy alone is in the region of 40–45% [1,2]. A number of randomized controlled trials have explored the role of chemotherapy prior to definitive local treatment (cystectomy or radiotherapy) of muscle invasive bladder cancer.

The largest of these is the European Organisation for Research and Treatment of Cancer/Medical Research Council (EORTC/MRC) trial of neoadjuvant chemotherapy. This trial included 976 patients with stage T2 G3, T3, T4a, N0-X, M0 transitional cell carcinoma (TCC) of the bladder who were deemed suitable for local radical treatment with cystectomy or external beam radiotherapy [3]. Patients were randomized to neoadjuvant chemotherapy (three cycles of cisplatin, methotrexate and vinblastine, CMV) followed by radical local treatment, or to radical local treatment alone (cystectomy in 484, radiotherapy in 414 and combined radiotherapy and surgery treatment in 77). Approximately 80% of patients randomized to the chemotherapy arm received all three cycles. Overall chemotherapy related mortality was 1% (five patients). Pathological complete response rate was 33% following CMV chemotherapy. An updated analysis [4] with a median follow-up of seven years has demonstrated an improvement in overall survival from 50.0 to 56.5% ($p = 0.03$).

The Nordic collaborative group have completed two large randomized trials of cisplatin-based combination chemotherapy followed by cystectomy, and a combined analysis of these two studies has been published [5]. Six hundred and twenty patients were treated from 1985 to 1997 with combination chemotherapy (cisplatin/doxorubicin or cisplatin/methotrexate) followed by cystectomy or cystectomy alone. Patients in the first trial also received pre-operative radiotherapy (4 Gy × 5). After a median follow-up of 4.7 years, an improvement in overall survival with neoadjuvant chemotherapy was seen, with a hazard ratio of 0.80 (95% confidence interval 0.64–0.99). Five-year survival was 56% in the neoadjuvant chemotherapy group, compared with 48% in the cystectomy alone group.

A Phase III US inter-group study evaluated the role of neoadjuvant M-VAC chemotherapy in patients with locally advanced bladder cancer who were to be treated with radical cystectomy [2]. Over a period of 11 years, 307 patients with stage T2-T4a invasive bladder cancer were recruited from 126 centers. Patients were randomized to surgery alone ($n = 154$) or to three cycles of M-VAC chemotherapy prior to surgery ($n = 153$). Patients were stratified according to age and stage and had to be of good performance status. At five years, 85% of patients with pT0 at the time of surgical resection were alive. Thirty-eight percent of patients who received M-VAC were found to have pT0 disease at the time of surgery, compared with 15% of patients in the surgery-alone group. An overall survival benefit was seen with neoadjuvant M-VAC chemotherapy (57% at five years compared with 43% in the surgery-alone group, $p = 0.06$). Neither tumor stage nor age had a significant interaction with treatment.

A meta-analysis first published in 2003 and updated in 2005 analyzed data for 3005 patients from 11 randomized trials, comparing neoadjuvant chemotherapy followed by either surgery or radiotherapy. Platinum-based combination chemotherapy demonstrated an overall survival benefit irrespective of local definitive treatment. The combined hazard ratio for combination chemotherapy was 0.86 (95% CI 0.77–0.95, $p = 0.003$). This is equivalent to a 5% absolute survival benefit at five years. An improvement in disease-free survival was also seen with platinum-based combination chemotherapy (HR = 0.78 95% CI 0.71–0.86, $p < 0.0001$), equivalent to a 9% absolute improvement at five years [1,6].

Summary

Cisplatin-based combination neoadjuvant chemotherapy in patients with muscle invasive disease appears to confer a survival benefit over local definitive treatment alone. At present, there is insufficient data to allow risk stratification according to stage of disease and patient characteristics.

Concurrent chemotherapy with radiotherapy

Chemotherapy with radiotherapy may have two potential benefits: first, as a radiosensitizer with the aim of improving the therapeutic ratio of radiotherapy, and second, to treat micrometastatic disease. Cisplatin has been shown to enhance the radiation effect in vivo, in vitro and under hypoxic conditions. The addition of cisplatin to radiotherapy has been shown to improve local control and survival in the management of cervical carcinoma and head and neck cancers [7–9]. A number of Phase II studies of concomitant chemotherapy have been published, with cisplatin, 5-FU and mitomycin C being the agents most commonly employed. Complete response rates of approximately 70% are reported [10–12]. The only randomized trial to date was performed by the National Cancer Institute of Canada, who conducted a prospective study of radiotherapy ± cisplatin in patients who were to receive radical local therapy (radiotherapy followed by cystectomy or definitive radiotherapy). This was a small study of 99 patients but showed that pelvic recurrence was found to be lower in patients who received cisplatin plus radiotherapy (absolute risk reduction of 20%). A trend toward lower rate of metastases free and overall survival was observed but the small size of this study meant these results were not statistically significant [10]. Many patients are unable to tolerate cisplatin because of their performance status or renal function. For this reason, the 5-FU/Mitomycin C is being explored in the UK in a Cancer Research UK-sponsored Phase III trial of radiotherapy with and without chemotherapy (BC2001). This trial is expected to close in late 2007.

Summary

Concurrent chemotherapy and radiotherapy has been demonstrated to be safe and effective with complete response rates of up to 70%. The optimal chemotherapy schedule and timing is yet to be defined.

Adjuvant chemotherapy

The benefit of adjuvant chemotherapy over neoadjuvant chemotherapy is that definitive local therapy is not delayed. Furthermore, accurate pathological staging data is possible following immediate cystectomy, and may allow risk stratification to determine those patients in whom chemotherapy may be more beneficial. On the other hand many patients take a considerable time to recover from surgery and only a proportion of patients are fit enough, or willing, to undergo this form of treatment within a reasonable time frame. These issues have made randomized clinical trials difficult to complete, with most trials being of small size, sometimes prematurely closed and with other methodological difficulties. Up to 25% of patients randomized to receive adjuvant chemotherapy did not receive any chemotherapy, or had significant protocol violations. Salvage chemotherapy regimens were not always specified for the control arm, and some trials were stopped early because of an apparent improvement at interim analysis. The evidence base for adjuvant chemotherapy is therefore less robust than that for neoadjuvant treatment. One metaanalysis has been published which has included individual patient data from 491 patients from six trials [13]. The authors acknowledge that the power of this metaanalysis is limited as only 66% of patients from all eligible trials were included. The hazard ratio for overall survival was 0.75 (95% confidence interval 0.60–0.96, $p = 0.019$) in favor of adjuvant chemotherapy.

Summary

Trials in the use of adjuvant chemotherapy following an attempt at definitive local treatment have tended to be small and underpowered and some have had flawed methodology. A metaanalysis suggests a possible survival advantage to adjuvant chemotherapy, but the authors conclude there is still insufficient evidence on which to base treatment decisions [13]. The EORTC 30994 trial of immediate versus delayed chemotherapy (classical M-VAC, high dose M-VAC or gemcitabine–cisplatin) after local treatment is currently accruing. This trial may go some way to answering these uncertainties.

Management of locally advanced disease and metastatic disease with palliative chemotherapy

Up to 50% of patients with muscle invasion at presentation will develop metastatic disease. Independent prognostic factors for survival include site of metastases and performance status. Patients with visceral metastases have a poorer prognosis than those with nodal disease. Karnofsky performance status less than 80% is also an adverse prognostic factor [14]. Systemic chemotherapy is usually considered for most patients with advanced bladder cancer who are fit enough to receive this treatment. A substantial proportion of patients have a poor performance status, or impaired organ function, and careful analysis of the risks versus benefit of treatment is important.

Single agent chemotherapy is effective, with response rates of between 15 and 20%, but with limited duration of response [15–18]. With the use of combination chemotherapy regimens, an increased response rate and survival has been achieved. The most commonly used schedules have historically been CMV [19] or M-VAC [16,20,21], which comprises methotrexate, vincristine and cisplatin with or without doxorubicin. Response rates of up to 50% have been reported, with complete response rates of approximately 10%. Progression-free survival rates with combination chemotherapy are in the region of seven to ten months compared with four months with single agent cisplatin [16]. The cost of such treatment is the considerable level of toxicity seen; for example, with M-VAC the following toxicities are reported, mucositis (49%), renal toxicity, febrile neutropenia (25%) and a toxic death rate of 3% [21].

Current research efforts are being directed to improve the cost–benefit ratio of bladder cancer chemotherapy. This could be achieved either by delivering improved efficacy or by delivering similar efficacy with a more favorable toxicity profile. Two regimes have been reported in recent years which on this basis seem to be improvements over the older schedules.

One schedule has used granulocyte colony-stimulating factors to accelerate the delivery of M-VAC with the aim of improving response rates and survival of patients with metastatic disease [22,23]. This accelerated schedule omits the day-15 and day-22 treatments (Table 8.1) and uses G-CSF to repeat the main drugs every 14 days. This accelerated M-VAC regimen has been compared to standard M-VAC in one randomized trial performed by the EORTC [24,25]. In this trial, 263 patients were randomized to receive accelerated M-VAC (two-weekly with G-CSF support) or standard M-VAC. There was an increased response rate in the experimental arm (CR 21% versus 12%) and an improvement in five-year survival (21.8% versus 13.5%). This improvement in survival did not, however, reach statistical significance. Perhaps counter-intuitively, this accelerated regime proved also to be less toxic and better tolerated than the standard schedule. This may be because of the low rate of neutropenia owing to routine G-CSF use and omitting extra methotrexate which could have caused a significant amount of the mucositis. This improvement in complete response rates and lowered toxicity is encouraging. Accelerated M-VAC is a particularly attractive chemotherapy schedule for neoadjuvant chemotherapy prior to definitive local treatment, in view of its efficacy and the short delivery time.

The alternative route to improve treatment is to explore newer chemotherapy agents, usually in combination with cisplatin. Gemcitabine and the taxanes (docetaxel and paclitaxel) have been of particular interest. Phase II studies have demonstrated response rates of approximately 50% to docetaxel and cisplatin in chemo-naïve patients [26,27]. Paclitaxel and carboplatin have been used in patients with renal impairment (which would preclude use of cisplatin) and response with rates of 24% and a median overall survival of 7.1 months [28]. Phase III data for taxanes is limited, but what is available is disappointing. One trial has demonstrated paclitaxel/carboplatin is a less toxic regimen than M-VAC. Firm conclusions with regard to the effect on survival are difficult as this trial failed to reach its accrual goal [29]. A Phase III trial of docetaxel/cisplatin (DC) has found that DC is inferior to M-VAC in terms of response, time to progression and survival [30]. Paclitaxel has also been used as second-line chemotherapy with reported response rates of 36% and a median time to progression of 6.2 months [31]. The other drug extensively studied is gemcitabine. Gemcitabine has single agent response rates in the order of 20–30% [32]. Gemcitabine and cisplatin in combination have been extensively studied in the Phase II setting, with response rates in the order of 40–60% [33,34]. One large randomized Phase III trial has compared this regimen with standard M-VAC. In this study, 405 patients with locally advanced or metastatic disease were randomly assigned to gemcitabine/cisplatin (GC) or M-VAC. Median survival was similar in both arms (14.0 months for GC versus 15.2 months for M-VAC). Five-year overall survival rates were not statistically different (13% for GC and 15.3% for M-VAC, $p = 0.53$). The toxicity profile of GC was improved, and more patients fared better with regard to weight, performance status and fatigue with GC [35,36], as well as less time in hospital and diminished use of antibiotics and other supportive treatments [37]. Gemcitabine and cisplatin have now been adopted as standard of care by many centers.

The most recent efforts have seen paclitaxel combined with GC in a triplet regimen. Impressive Phase II results have been reported (response rate 78%; median survival 24 months) [38]. This schedule has been tested in a large EORTC Phase III trial against GC. Results are currently awaited.

A significant proportion of patients have poor renal function or a poor perfor-mance status, which would preclude treatment with cisplatin. Management of these patients can be difficult. Some patients can be treated with fractionated cisplatin over two days [12] or by using the cisplatin analogue, carboplatin. Carboplatin is an active agent in bladder cancer, but the overall efficacy may be less [39]. Patients with more extensive disease and poorer performance status have a significantly poorer survival [40]. The value of chemotherapy in this setting remains debatable and requires careful discussion with the patient. If used, suitable treatments would be gemcitabine 1000 mg/m^2 day-1 and day-8 combined with carboplatin AUC 4.5[1] repeated every three weeks or single agent gemcitabine 1250 mg/m^2 day-1 and day-8.

Patient care during chemotherapy

In view of the potential toxicity with bladder chemotherapy, careful monitoring is required during treatment for toxicity and response. In most instances, patients are seen weekly to monitor hematological, liver and renal function as well as to undertake toxicity assessment, looking particularly for fatigue, mucositis, gastro-intestinal upset (nausea, vomiting, constipation or diarrhea) and peripheral neu-ropathy. Treatment-related renal impairment is common, often because of the effects of cisplatin. It is important to avoid dehydration, and admission for intravenous rehydration may be required if patients are unable to maintain an adequate fluid intake. Renal obstruction may occur, and should be excluded if renal function deteriorates. Particular care has to be taken when using methotrex-ate, which is renally excreted. In patients with renal insufficiency or with third space fluid (ascites, pleural effusion and edema), methotrexate can accumulate and lead to life-threatening toxicities such as mucositis and bone marrow suppression. In such cases, plasma methotrexate levels should be monitored and folinic acid rescue employed. Other drugs such as adriamycin, gemcitabine and taxanes are excreted via the liver and should be used with care if there is liver impairment. Patients developing significant hematological toxicity should usually undergo dose reduction or have G-CSF commenced. The risk of neutropenic sepsis may be reduced by using prophylactic antibiotics [41].

[1.] AUC = Area under the curve. This is used to calculate carboplatin dose according to the Calvert formula; Dose = AUC × (GFR + 25).

Most available data would suggest that only patients attaining a good clinical response to treatment gain symptomatic and survival benefit [42]. We would therefore advise that early response assessment after two cycles (or at most three cycles) be undertaken by repeating cross-sectional imaging. Non-responding patients should stop treatment and consider alternative management strategies, whereas responding patients complete the usual treatment course of six cycles of therapy. Intermediate cross-sectional imaging is often undertaken to confirm response is being maintained. There is little data to suggest that extending treatment beyond six cycles improves outcome and such treatment only adds to cumulative toxicity. Many tumors can secrete tumor markers such as HCG, Ca19-9, CEA and Ca-125. Though not well validated, these markers may help guide response assessment, as changes in markers may mirror and pre-date imaging changes [43].

Summary

Combination chemotherapy leads to improved survival over single agent chemotherapy in patients with advanced and metastatic bladder cancer. Median survival with treatment is now in the region of 12–13 months. A combination of gemcitabine and cisplatin appears to be as effective as standard M-VAC chemotherapy but with less toxicity. In patients with renal insufficiency carboplatin can be substituted for cisplatin.

REFERENCES

1. Advanced Bladder Cancer Meta-analysis Collaboration. Neoadjuvant chemotherapy in invasive bladder cancer: a systematic review and meta-analysis. *Lancet* 2003; **361**: 1927–34.
2. Grossman H B, Natale R B, Tangen C M *et al.* Neoadjuvant chemotherapy plus cystectomy compared with cystectomy alone for locally advanced bladder cancer. *N Engl J Med* 2003; **349**: 859–66.
3. International Collaboration of Trialists. Neoadjuvant cisplatin, methotrexate, and vinblastine chemotherapy for muscle-invasive bladder cancer: a randomised controlled trial. *Lancet* 1999; **354**: 533–40.
4. Hall R. On behalf of the International Collaboration of Trialists of the MRC Bladder Cancer Group; MRC Clinical Trials Unit, UK: Updated results of a randomised controlled trial of

neoadjuvant cisplatin (C) methotrexate (M) and vinblastine (V) for muscle-invasive bladder cancer. In: *Proceedings of the American Society of Clinical Oncology*, Thirty-Eighth Annual Meeting, 2002; Orlando, Florida.

5. Sherif A, Holmberg L, Rintala E *et al*. Neoadjuvant cisplatinum based combination chemotherapy in patients with invasive bladder cancer: a combined analysis of two Nordic studies. *Eur Urol* 2004; **45**: 297–303.

6. Advanced Bladder Cancer (ABC) Meta-analysis Collaboration. Neoadjuvant chemotherapy in invasive bladder cancer: update of a systematic review and meta-analysis of individual patient data advanced bladder cancer (ABC) meta-analysis collaboration. *Eur Urol* 2005; **48**: 202–5; discussion 205–6.

7. Pearcey R, Brundage M, Drouin P *et al*. Phase III trial comparing radical radiotherapy with and without cisplatin chemotherapy in patients with advanced squamous cell cancer of the cervix. *J Clin Oncol* 2002; **20**: 966–72.

8. Pignon J P, Bourhis J, Domenge C, Designe L. Chemotherapy added to locoregional treatment for head and neck squamous-cell carcinoma: three meta-analyses of updated individual data. MACH-NC Collaborative Group. Meta-analysis of chemotherapy on head and neck cancer. *Lancet* 2000; **355**: 949–55.

9. Rose P G, Bundy B N, Watkins E B *et al*. Concurrent cisplatin-based radiotherapy and chemotherapy for locally advanced cervical cancer. *N Engl J Med* 1999; **340**: 1144–53.

10. Coppin C M, Gospodarowicz M K, James K *et al*. Improved local control of invasive bladder cancer by concurrent cisplatin and preoperative or definitive radiation. The National Cancer Institute of Canada Clinical Trials Group. *J Clin Oncol* 1996; **14**: 2901–7.

11. Gogna N K, Matthews J H, Turner S L *et al*. Efficacy and tolerability of concurrent weekly low dose cisplatin during radiation treatment of localized muscle invasive bladder transitional cell carcinoma: a report of two sequential Phase II studies from the Trans Tasman Radiation Oncology Group. *Radiother Oncol* 2006; **81**: 9–17.

12. Hussain S A, Stocken D D, Riley P *et al*. A phase I/II study of gemcitabine and fractionated cisplatin in an outpatient setting using a 21-day schedule in patients with advanced and metastatic bladder cancer. *Br J Cancer* 2004; **91**: 844–9.

13. Advanced Bladder Cancer (ABC) Meta-analysis Collaboration. Adjuvant chemotherapy in invasive bladder cancer: a systematic review and meta-analysis of individual patient data Advanced Bladder Cancer (ABC) Meta-analysis Collaboration. *Eur Urol* 2005; **48**: 189–99; discussion 199–201.

14. Bajorin D F, Dodd P M, Mazumdar M *et al*. Long-term survival in metastatic transitional-cell carcinoma and prognostic factors predicting outcome of therapy. *J Clin Oncol* 1999; **17**: 3173–81.

15. Hillcoat B L, Raghavan D, Matthews J *et al*. A randomized trial of cisplatin versus cisplatin plus methotrexate in advanced cancer of the urothelial tract. *J Clin Oncol* 1989; **7**: 706–9.

16. Loehrer P J, Sr., Einhorn L H, Elson P J *et al*. A randomized comparison of cisplatin alone or in combination with methotrexate, vinblastine, and doxorubicin in patients with metastatic urothelial carcinoma: a cooperative group study. *J Clin Oncol* 1992; **10**: 1066–73.

17. Papamichael D, Gallagher C J, Oliver R T *et al*. Phase II study of paclitaxel in pretreated patients with locally advanced/metastatic cancer of the bladder and ureter. *Br J Cancer* 1997; **75**: 606–7.

18. Yang M H, Yen C C, Chang Y H *et al*. Single agent paclitaxel as a first-line therapy in advanced urothelial carcinoma: its efficacy and safety in patients even with pretreatment renal insufficiency. *Jpn J Clin Oncol* 2000; **30**: 547–52.

19. Harker W G, Meyers F J, Freiha F S *et al*. Cisplatin, methotrexate, and vinblastine (CMV): an effective chemotherapy regimen for metastatic transitional cell carcinoma of the urinary tract. A Northern California Oncology Group study. *J Clin Oncol* 1985; **3**: 1463–70.

20. Sternberg C N, Yagoda A, Scher H I. Chemotherapy for advanced urothelial tract tumors: the M-VAC regimen. *Prog Clin Biol Res* 1988; **277**: 45–51.

21. Sternberg C N, Yagoda A, Scher H I *et al*. Methotrexate, vinblastine, doxorubicin, and cisplatin for advanced transitional cell carcinoma of the urothelium. Efficacy and patterns of response and relapse. *Cancer* 1989; **64**: 2448–58.

22. Loehrer P J, Sr., Elson P, Dreicer R *et al*. Escalated dosages of methotrexate, vinblastine, doxorubicin, and cisplatin plus recombinant human granulocyte colony-stimulating factor in advanced urothelial carcinoma: an Eastern Cooperative Oncology Group trial. *J Clin Oncol* 1994; **12**: 483–8.

23. Sternberg C N, de Mulder P H, van Oosterom A T *et al*. Escalated M-VAC chemotherapy and recombinant human granulocyte-macrophage colony stimulating factor (rhGM-CSF) in patients with advanced urothelial tract tumors. *Ann Oncol* 1993; **4**: 403–7.

24. Sternberg C N, de Mulder P, Schornagel J H *et al*. Seven year update of an EORTC phase III trial of high-dose intensity M-VAC chemotherapy and G-CSF versus classic M-VAC in advanced urothelial tract tumours. *Eur J Cancer* 2006; **42**: 50–4.

25. Sternberg C N, de Mulder P H, Schornagel J H *et al*. Randomized phase III trial of high-dose-intensity methotrexate, vinblastine, doxorubicin, and cisplatin (MVAC) chemotherapy and recombinant human granulocyte colony-stimulating factor versus classic MVAC in advanced urothelial tract tumors: European Organization for Research and Treatment of Cancer Protocol no. 30924. *J Clin Oncol* 2001; **19**: 2638–46.

26. Dimopoulos M A, Bakoyannis C, Georgoulias V *et al*. Docetaxel and cisplatin combination chemotherapy in advanced carcinoma of the urothelium: a multicenter phase II study of the Hellenic Cooperative Oncology Group. *Ann Oncol* 1999; **10**: 1385–8.

27. Garcia del Muro X, Marcuello E, Guma J *et al*. Phase II multicentre study of docetaxel plus cisplatin in patients with advanced urothelial cancer. *Br J Cancer* 2002; **86**: 326–30.

28. Vaughn D J, Manola J, Dreicer R *et al*. Phase II study of paclitaxel plus carboplatin in patients with advanced carcinoma of the urothelium and renal dysfunction (E2896): a trial of the Eastern Cooperative Oncology Group. *Cancer* 2002; **95**: 1022–7.

29. Dreicer R, Manola J, Roth B J *et al*. Phase III trial of methotrexate, vinblastine, doxorubicin, and cisplatin versus carboplatin and paclitaxel in patients with advanced carcinoma of the urothelium. *Cancer* 2004; **100**: 1639–45.

30. Bamias A, Aravantinos G, Deliveliotis C *et al.* Docetaxel and cisplatin with granulocyte colony-stimulating factor (G-CSF) versus MVAC with G-CSF in advanced urothelial carcinoma: a multicenter, randomized, phase III study from the Hellenic Cooperative Oncology Group. *J Clin Oncol* 2004; **22**: 220–8.

31. Uhm J E, Lim H Y, Kim W S *et al.* Paclitaxel with cisplatin as salvage treatment for patients with previously treated advanced transitional cell carcinoma of the urothelial tract. *Neoplasia* 2007; **9**: 18–22.

32. Lorusso V, Pollera C F, Antimi M *et al.* A phase II study of gemcitabine in patients with transitional cell carcinoma of the urinary tract previously treated with platinum. Italian Co-operative Group on Bladder Cancer. *Eur J Cancer* 1998; **34**: 1208–12.

33. Moore M J, Winquist E W, Murray N *et al.* Gemcitabine plus cisplatin, an active regimen in advanced urothelial cancer: a phase II trial of the National Cancer Institute of Canada Clinical Trials Group. *J Clin Oncol* 1999; **17**: 2876–81.

34. von der Maase H, Andersen L, Crino L *et al.* Weekly gemcitabine and cisplatin combination therapy in patients with transitional cell carcinoma of the urothelium: a phase II clinical trial. *Ann Oncol* 1999; **10**: 1461–5.

35. von der Maase H, Hansen S W, Roberts J T *et al.* Gemcitabine and cisplatin versus methotrexate, vinblastine, doxorubicin, and cisplatin in advanced or metastatic bladder cancer: results of a large, randomized, multinational, multicenter, phase III study. *J Clin Oncol* 2000; **18**: 3068–77.

36. von der Maase H, Sengelov L, Roberts J T *et al.* Long-term survival results of a randomized trial comparing gemcitabine plus cisplatin, with methotrexate, vinblastine, doxorubicin, plus cisplatin in patients with bladder cancer. *J Clin Oncol* 2005; **23**: 4602–8.

37. Von der Maase H, Hansen S W, Liepa A *et al.* Health care resource use for patients with advanced bladder cancer treated with gemcitabine plus cisplatin (GC) versus MVAC in a phase III trial. *Ann Oncol* 2000; **11**(suppl 4): 74 (abst 3270).

38. Bellmunt J, Guillem V, Paz-Ares L *et al.* Phase I-II study of paclitaxel, cisplatin, and gemcitabine in advanced transitional-cell carcinoma of the urothelium. Spanish Oncology Genitourinary Group. *J Clin Oncol* 2000; **18**: 3247–55.

39. Bellmunt J, Ribas A, Eres N *et al.* Carboplatin-based versus cisplatin-based chemotherapy in the treatment of surgically incurable advanced bladder carcinoma. *Cancer* 1997; **80**: 1966–72.

40. Mead G M, Russell M, Clark P *et al.* A randomized trial comparing methotrexate and vinblastine (MV) with cisplatin, methotrexate and vinblastine (CMV) in advanced transitional cell carcinoma: results and a report on prognostic factors in a Medical Research Council study. MRC Advanced Bladder Cancer Working Party. *Br J Cancer* 1998; **78**: 1067–75.

41. Cullen M, Steven N, Billingham L *et al.* Antibacterial prophylaxis after chemotherapy for solid tumors and lymphomas. *N Engl J Med* 2005; **353**: 988–98.

42. Fossa S D, Sternberg C, Scher H I *et al.* Survival of patients with advanced urothelial cancer treated with cisplatin-based chemotherapy. *Br J Cancer* 1996; **74**: 1655–9.

43. Cook A M, Huddart R A, Jay G *et al.* The utility of tumour markers in assessing the response to chemotherapy in advanced bladder cancer. *Br J Cancer* 2000; **82**: 1952–7.

9

Clinical follow-up of bladder cancer

Alan Thompson and Sarb Sandhu

Superficial bladder cancer

Cystoscopic follow-up

There is no doubt that cystoscopy remains the gold standard of follow-up for patients who have undergone a transurethral resection (TUR) of a superficial bladder cancer. The majority will undergo a flexible cystoscopy, which obviates the need for a general or spinal anesthetic and which is very well tolerated. A flexible cystoscopy allows the regular inspection of the urethra and the whole bladder with a low morbidity and low cost. With modern videocystoscopes and experience, even very small recurrences can be readily detected. The interpretation of flat mucosal lesions is, however, difficult.

The first check cystoscopy is performed three months following the initial TUR apart from in those cases where there is a question over the grade (G2 or G3) or when there is uncertainity as to the depth of invasion of the tumor. In such cases, an early repeat resection or biopsy is made at the site of the initial tumor (4–6 weeks) [1]. However, although some doubt that the repeat early TUR has any effect on the subsequent outcome of these cases, it has been shown to reduce recurrences and improve prognosis. Indeed, there is a 10% chance that a G3TaT1 tumor has been understaged and is therefore a muscle invasive tumor [1–3]. The treatment of muscle invasive bladder tumors is completely different to that of superficial bladder tumors (see Chapter 6).

There are two main questions regarding the follow-up of patients after treatment for superficial bladder cancer. These are
1. At what sort of frequency should follow-up occur?
2. How long should follow-up be continued?

Carcinoma of the Bladder, ed. David MacVicar. Published by Cambridge University Press. © Cambridge University Press 2008.

There have been several studies that have investigated the factors that may predict recurrence and define patients requiring further treatment. Two of the largest series are those of the Medical Research Council (MRC) and of the European Organisation for Research and Treatment for Cancer (EORTC) [4,5]. These are based on patients entered into their randomized trials of intravesical chemotherapy. In these studies, only patients fulfilling the entry criteria for the intravesical chemotherapy studies are included and so generalizations from this data must be interpreted with care. Both studies highlighted the importance of grade of tumor as well as the number of tumors at presentation. The three-month cystoscopy findings were also found to be a predictor of subsequent recurrence. Indeed, in the MRC analysis, if the results from the three-month cystoscopy were combined with the number of tumors at presentation, no other factor added significantly to the prediction of recurrence. Not surprisingly, disease recurrence at cystoscopy continues to be highly predictive of future recurrence, with the probability of developing recurrence decreasing with each negative cystoscopy. In all studies, the numbers of patients getting a tumor recurrence are highest in the first two years, reaching 8% at five years and 0% at 10 years [6]. In these studies, T stage (Ta v T1) was not strong a predictor for recurrence but it is likely that T stage does predict for risk of progression, as shown by Kurth *et al.* [5].

Therefore, follow-up regimens are designed to take this into account. The European Association of Urology (EAU) guidelines for cystoscopic review are based on placing patients into three risk categories [7] as follows.

Low risk

G1Ta tumors (approximately 50% of all patients), usually single and less than 3 cm, should have the first check cystoscopy at three months. If negative, the next cystoscopy should be at nine months and if this is clear then subsequent cystoscopies should be yearly.

High risk

G3Ta/T1 and G2Ta/T1 multiple tumors and those greater than 3 cm (approximately 15% of all patients) should have a cystoscopy at three-monthly intervals for two years, if clear at the first check, followed by four-monthly in the third year, six-monthly until year 5 and then annually thereafter.

Intermediate risk

Such patients fall between the other two groups and should be offered a schedule that lies in-between the low-risk and high-risk groups. In the case of disease recurrence, the histological findings are the same as those of the primary TUR in over 95% of cases.

The question of duration of follow-up depends largely upon the natural history of the disease in an individual patient. If a recurrence is found at cystoscopy then the schedule reverts back to the beginning for deciding on subsequent surveillance. It has been suggested that in the low-risk group the period of surveillance could end at five years, with the high-risk group undergoing lifelong surveillance and the intermediate group continuing for ten years. However, there are reports of recurrences of superficial bladder cancer even after long, disease-free intervals, indicating a need for lifelong surveillance [8,9].

Patients with regular recurrences will continue to have them until death or progression and the need for radical treatment. Patients with recurrences during the first four years after TUR continue to have lifelong recurrences [10].

In attempts to avoid cystoscopy, ultrasonography and more recently computed tomographic virtual cystoscopy have been used or suggested for the follow-up of superficial papillary bladder cancers. Although both can detect tumors of a few millimeters in diameter, neither is, as yet, proven to be as reliable as cystoscopy and both preclude the acquisition of tissue for histology [11,12]. In the case of virtual cystoscopy, there is also the additional concern of exposure to radiation.

Urine cytology

The sensitivity of voided urine cytology varies from 25% for low-grade lesions to 76% for high-grade lesions, which reduces its value as a surveillance marker [13,14]. However, its use as part of disease surveillance is justified because of the high specificity (98–100%) and relatively high sensitivity in high-grade tumors.

In response to these limitations, a number of new diagnostic tests have been developed to detect tumor-specific antigens in voided urine. Examples of these include tests to determine expression of nuclear matrix proteins, Lewis X antigen expression on exfoliated urothelial cells and telomerase activity in exfoliated cells. The clinical utility of these new tumor markers is, however, not established in the routine follow-up of bladder cancer [15–17].

Upper tract surveillance – IVU

It is rare to develop an upper tract tumor during follow-up for superficial bladder cancer and so the routine requesting of regular intravenous urography (IVU) as part of follow-up is not necessary [18]. However, in patients with high-risk tumors, and especially those with carcinoma *in situ* (CIS), or in patients with unexplained positive cytology, upper tract surveillance is recommended [19,20]. It may also have its uses in selected patients such as heavy smokers, industrial workers exposed to known carcinogens and patients with vesicoureteric reflux, all of which are well-established risk factors for development of urothelial tumors.

Muscle invasive bladder cancer

Cancer follow-up after radical surgery

The purpose of following up patients with invasive bladder cancer after radical exenterative surgery (and radiotherapy) is to detect the presence of local or distant recurrences as early as possible in order to be able to offer additional treatment when indicated. It is evident that patients who have a symptomatic evidence of recurrence/progression also have a poor performance status and are less likely to be able to tolerate adjuvant treatment [21].

The follow-up schedule following radical cystectomy for muscle invasive bladder cancer is very much directed by the risk of tumor progression and the anatomical sites of progression or relapse. The risk of tumor progression following a radical cystectomy is dependent upon the pathological stage. The tumors are always high grade or carcinoma *in situ*. The risk of tumor progression decreases from almost 100% in patients with pN2 disease down to 5% in patients having primary radical surgery for G3pT1 disease [22,23].

As in superficial bladder cancer, where the risk of recurrence is highest in the first two years, so in muscle invasive bladder cancer the risk of progression or relapse is highest in the first two years. The risks become relatively low after three years.

New tumors may occur in the remnants of the urinary tract such as the urethra and the upper tract (ureters and renal pelvis). The risk of detecting new tumors in the urothelial remnants (5–15%) does not decrease with time. Approximately half of all cases occur within the first 12 months [24,25]. The majority of cases occur in the male urethra in cases where it is not removed at the time of the original surgery (5–12%) [26,27]. As this risk does not decrease with time, the patient is effectively considered to be always at high risk of recurrence. Examination of the urethra, either by endoscopy or by cytology following lavage with saline, should be lifelong. Although upper tract tumors are found infrequently after cystectomy, they are often advanced when detected [28]. This and the need to survey the upper tracts for ureteric dilatation because of stenosis or stricture make upper tract imaging useful after cystectomy.

Tumor progression may be local, in regional lymph nodes or as distant metastatic spread. Of all cases of relapse after surgery 15–20% occur locally in the true pelvis, while another 10–15% occur in the pelvic and retroperitoneal lymph nodes. Therefore, cross-sectional imaging of the abdomen and pelvis will detect up to 35% of all cases of progression.

While distant metastatic disease can be found in any organ, lung, bone and liver are the commonest sites (see Chapter 5). More than 50% of patients who progress will do so with distant metastatic disease. Therefore, it would seem sensible to add cross-sectional imaging of the chest to that of the abdomen and pelvis. This, if combined with a bone scan, will detect 85% of all cases of progressive disease. As with other solid tumors, there is limited evidence that surveillance for asymptomatic metastatic disease contributes positively to survival.

Consequences of a urinary diversion

There are a number of consequences to having a urinary diversion. These can be broadly categorized as metabolic, dependent on the nature of the bowel segment used, those owing to the surgery itself, infections and less commonly the risk of second malignancies.

Metabolic consequences of urinary diversion

As the function of the bowel varies with each part of the bowel, the metabolic consequences are very dependent on the type and length of bowel used to create the conduit or reservoir. Using the terminal ileum will result in vitamin B12 deficiency that may not become apparent for a number of years (depending on the amount of vitamin B12 stored in the body) [29]. Ileo-cecal resections are twice as likely to cause chronic diarrhea than the use of ileum alone. The resection of more than 60 cm of ileum may lead to problems involving bile and fatty acid absorption.

Continent diversions, reservoirs rather than conduits, allow the absorption of urine electrolytes. The resorption of the urinary electrolytes must be balanced by adequate renal function in order to try to maintain a normal electrolyte and acid–base balance. The degree of absorption is dependent upon the type of bowel used to form the reservoir, the surface area of the reservoir in contact with the urine and also the dwell time (the time that the urine is in contact with the absorptive surface of the reservoir). Ileal segments have a greater tendency to absorb sodium than colonic segments, whereas conversely colonic segments tend to absorb more chloride. Consequently, colonic reservoirs are more likely to lead to a metabolic hyperchloremic acidosis, although up to 50% of ileal reservoirs are found to have a mild acidosis principally owing to the absorption of ammonia [30,31].

Irrespective of the bowel segment used, all continent reservoirs are known to lead to increased losses of calcium, magnesium and phosphate, leading to the theoretical risk, at least, of problems with bone demineralization [32].

As well as the absorption of urinary electrolytes, continent diversions also absorb a significant amount of fluid, which may have an impact upon fluid balance.

Complications of surgery

The specific complications common to all types of urinary diversion, continent or otherwise, are ureteric strictures and reflux. Surgical technique as well as tissue quality, i.e. whether there has been previous irradiation, will influence the frequency of these complications.

Ileal conduits are prone to elongation, stomal stenosis, parastomal herniation as well as the above [29,33]. Continent reservoirs may have problems related to the continence mechanism, e.g. problems with catheterization or leakage from a Mitrofanoff procedure may occur. Urethral stenosis, incontinence (especially night time in 20–30% of patients) and failure to void (30% in females) are all seen after orthotopic bladder substitution [34].

Infections

There is little data on the true incidence of bacteriuria in patients who have undergone a urinary diversion. Bacteria can be commonly found in the urine from patients with ileal conduits, but in the majority this appears to be of little consequence [35,36]. Pyelonephritis and hematuria tend to be the most common sequelae in those patients in whom it causes problems.

Infection in the presence of metabolic disorders does lead to stone formation. This is more likely to occur in continent diversions and has been reported to be as high as 34% at five years in some series [37,38].

Second malignancies

Second malignancies, unrelated to the cause of the primary, are known to develop after urinary diversions. They are most likely to occur at the junction between the ureter and the bowel at the site of the anastomosis and histologically are usually adenocarcinomas. It is thought that nitrosamine production, owing to the presence of bacteria and in the presence of a metabolic disorder, may lead to the development of these tumors. There is a long latent period before the development of such tumors, usually more than 20 years, but tumors have been reported as early as five years [39,40].

With these consequences of urinary diversion in mind, follow-up protocols should include regular estimations of electrolyte levels and acid–base balance. Some form of imaging, dependent on that used for cancer follow-up, will need to be used to exclude stone formation. The pouch should be visually inspected by means of yearly endoscopy, up to five years from the time of the original cystectomy.

Follow-up after radical radiotherapy

It is essential to follow up the bladders in patients who have been treated with radiotherapy for muscle invasive bladder cancer indefinitely. This is usually achieved by cystoscopic review as well as urine cytology. Superficial recurrences in the bladder are managed in a similar way to managing those in patients who have not had radiotherapy: by a combination of transurethral resection and additional intravesical therapy (chemo- or immunotherapy) as dictated by the grade and stage of the recurrence. In the case of invasive recurrences, salvage cystectomy should be performed where possible and in the absence of metastatic disease.

Follow-up aimed at detecting metastatic disease is along the same principles as for patients who have undergone radical curative surgical procedures.

Conclusion

The treatment of superficial bladder cancer is relatively straightforward, being mainly endoscopic with the use of intravesical agents when necessary. It is not surprising, therefore, that the cystoscopic follow-up of superficial bladder cancer is well established. Schedules of follow-up are based on large-scale studies, with the MRC and EORTC studies being two of the largest. As such, the frequency of cystoscopic review can be tailored, based on the likelihood of recurrence and the necessity of further treatment. Similarly, frequency of upper tract surveillance in superficial disease is relatively well established. Conversely, in muscle invasive bladder cancer, which comprises only approximately 15% of newly diagnosed bladder cancers, radical treatments are far more varied. Surgical approaches, with or without urinary diversions, are variable; radiotherapy, chemotherapy or combinations of these are also therapeutic options. There are no large-scale studies comparing follow-up schedules in these clinical circumstances, and in such cases follow-up is based on the likelihood of recurrence or progression of the cancer, the consequences of the treatment given and the development of new symptoms.

REFERENCES

1. Schwaibold H E, Sivalingam S, May F, Hartung R. The value of a second transurethral resection for T1 bladder cancer. *BJU Int* 2006; **97**: 1199–201.
2. Miladi M, Peyromaure M, Zerbib M *et al*. The value of a second transurethral resection in evaluating patients with bladder tumours. *Eur Urol* 2003; **43**: 241–5.
3. Jakse G, Algaba F, Malmstrom P U, Oosterlinck W. A second-look TUR in T1 transitional cell carcinoma: why? *Eur Urol* 2004; **45**: 539–46.
4. Parmar M K, Freedman L S, Hargreave T B, Tolley D A. Prognostic factors for recurrence and follow-up policies in the treatment of superficial bladder cancer: report from the British Medical Research Council Subgroup on Superfical Bladder Cancer (Urological Cancer Working Party). *J Urol* 1989; **142**: 284–8.
5. Kurth K H, Denis L, Bouffioux C *et al*. Factors affecting recurrence and progression in superficial bladder tumours. *Eur J Cancer* 1995; **31A**: 1840–6.
6. Fitzpatrick J M, West A B, Butler M R *et al*. Superficial bladder tumours (stage pTa, grades 1 and 2): the importance of recurrence pattern following initial resection. *J Urol* 1986; **135**: 920–2.
7. Oosterlinck W, van der Meijden A, Sylvester R *et al*. *Guidelines on TaT1 (non-muscle invasive) Bladder Cancer (update)*. European Association of Urology Guidelines; March 2006. ISBN: 90-70244-37-3 (http://www.uroweb.org/nc/professional-resources/guidelines/online)
8. Morris S B, Gordon E M, Shearer R J, Woodhouse C R. Superficial bladder cancer: for how long should a tumour-free patient have check cystoscopies? *Br J Urol* 1995; **75**: 193–6.
9. Thompson R A, Campbell E W, Kramer H C *et al*. Late invasive recurrence despite long-term surveillance for superficial bladder cancer. *J Urol* 1993; **149**: 1010–11.
10. Holmang S, Hedelin H, Anderstrom C, Johansson S L. The relationship among multiple recurrences, progression and prognosis of patients with stages Ta and T1 transitional cell cancer of the bladder followed for at least 20 years. *J Urol* 1995; **153**: 1823–7.

11. Olsen L H, Genster H G. Prolonging follow-up intervals for non-invasive bladder tumours: a randomized controlled trial. *Scand J Urol Nephrol Suppl* 1995; **172**: 33–6.

12. Tsili ACh, Tsampoulas C, Chatziparaskevas N *et al.* Computed tomographic virtual cystoscopy for the detection of urinary bladder neoplasms. *Eur Urol* 2004; **46**: 579–85.

13. Badalament R A, Hermansen D K, Kimmel M *et al.* The sensitivity of bladder wash flow cytometry, bladder wash cytology, and voided cytology in the detection of bladder carcinoma. *Cancer* 1987; **60**: 1423–7.

14. Badalament R A, Kimmel M, Gay H *et al.* The sensitivity of flow cytometry compared with conventional cytology in the detection of superficial bladder carcinoma. *Cancer* 1987; **59**: 2078–85.

15. Wiener H G, Mian C, Haitel A *et al.* Can urine bound diagnostic tests replace cystoscopy in the management of bladder cancer? *J Urol* 1998; **159**: 1876–80.

16. Golijanin D, Sherman Y, Shapiro A, Pode D. Detection of bladder tumours by immunostaining of the Lewis X antigen in cells from voided urine. *Urology* 1995; **46**: 173–7.

17. Yoshida K, Sugino T, Tahara H *et al.* Telomerase activity in bladder carcinoma and its implication for noninvasive diagnosis by detection of exfoliated cancer cells in urine. *Cancer* 1997; **79**: 362–9.

18. Holmang S, Hedelin H, Anderstrom C *et al.* Long-term follow-up of a bladder carcinoma cohort: routine follow-up urography is not necessary. *J Urol* 1998; **160**: 45–8.

19. Herr H W. Tumour progression and survival in patients with T1G3 bladder tumours: 15-year outcome. *Br J Urol* 1997; **80**: 762–5.

20. Miller E B, Eure G R, Schellhammer P F. Upper tract transitional cell carcinoma following treatment of superficial bladder cancer with BCG. *Urology* 1993; **42**: 26–30.

21. Sengelov L, Nielsen O S, Kamby C, von der Maase H. Platinum analogue combination chemotherapy: cisplatin, carboplatin, and methotrexate in patients with metastatic urothelial tract tumors. A phase II trial with evaluation of prognostic factors. *Cancer* 1995; **76**: 1797–803.

22. Ghoneim M A, el-Mekresh M M, el-Baz M A *et al.* Radical cystectomy for carcinoma of the bladder: critical evaluation of the results in 1,026 cases. *J Urol* 1997; **158**: 393–9.

23. Skinner D G, Lieskovsky G. Contemporary cystectomy with pelvic node dissection compared to preoperative radiation therapy plus cystectomy in management of invasive bladder cancer. *J Urol* 1984; **131**: 1069–72.

24. Beahrs J R, Fleming T R, Zincke H. Risk of local urethral recurrence after radical cystectomy for bladder cancer. *J Urol* 1984; **131**: 264–6.

25. Stöckle M, Gökcebay E, Riedmiller H, Hohenfellner R. Urethral tumor recurrences after radical cystoprostatectomy: the case for primary cystoprostatourethrectomy? *J Urol* 1990; **143**: 41–3.

26. Darson M F, Blute M B, Barrett D M. Continent orthotopic urinary diversion in female patients. *American Urological Association Update Series* 2000; **19**: 257–64.

27. Skinner D G, Stein J P, Lieskovsky G *et al.* 25-year experience in the management of invasive bladder cancer by radical cystectomy. *Eur Urol* 1998; **33**(suppl 4): 25–6.

28. Balaji K C, McGuire M, Grotas J et al. Upper tract recurrences following radical cystectomy: an analysis of prognostic factors, recurrence pattern and stage at presentation. *J Urol* 1999; **162**: 1603–6.

29. Sullivan J W, Grabstald H, Whitmore W F. Complications of ureteroileal conduit with radical cystectomy: review of 336 cases. *J Urol* 1980; **124**: 797–801.

30. Koch M O, McDougal W S. The pathophysiology of hypercloremic metabolic acidosis after urinary diversion through intestinal segments. *Surgery* 1985; **98**: 561–70.

31. Nurse D E, Mundy A R. Metabolic complication of cystoplasty. *Br J Urol* 1989; **63**: 165–70.

32. McDougal W S, Koch M O, Shands C 3rd, Price R R. Bony demineralization following urinary intestinal diversion. *J Urol* 1988; **140**: 853–5.

33. Wallace D M. Uretero-ileostomy. *Br J Urol* 1970; **42**: 529–34.

34. Whitmore W F 3rd, Gittes R F. Reconstruction of the urinary tract by cecal and ileocecal cystoplasty: review of a 15-year experience. *J Urol* 1983; **129**: 494–8.

35. Middleton A W Jr., Hendren W H. Ileal conduits in children at the Massachusetts General Hospital from 1955 to 1970. *J Urol* 1976; **115**: 591–5.

36. Elder D D, Moisey C U, Rees R W. A long-term follow-up of the colonic conduit operation in children. *Br J Urol* 1979; **51**: 462–5.

37. Terai A, Ueda T, Kakehi Y et al. Urinary calculi as a later complication of the Indiana continent urinary diversion: comparison with the Kock pouch procedure. *J Urol* 1996; **155**: 66–8.

38. Wilson T G, Moreno J G, Weinberg A, Ahlering T E. Late complications of the modified Indiana pouch. *J Urol* 1994; **151**: 331–4.

39. Schipper H, Decter A. Carcinoma of the colon arising at ureteral implant sites despite early external diversion: pathogenetic and clinical implications. *Cancer* 1981; **47**: 2062–5.

40. Stewart M, Macrae F A, Williams C B. Neoplasia and ureterosigmoidostomy: a colonoscopy survey. *Br J Surg* 1982; **69**: 414–16.

Imaging of treated bladder cancer

Ben Taylor, Suzanne Bonington and Bernadette Carrington

Imaging has a well-established role in the pre-treatment assessment of bladder cancer. Staging of muscle invasive tumors with CT or MRI is accurate and has an immediate effect on treatment decisions [1–3]. However, the role of imaging in monitoring the effects of treatment and in the follow-up of the treated patient is less well defined.

This chapter will consider the role of imaging in the diagnosis of treatment-related complications, the recognition of normal post-treatment tissue appearances and the assessment of treatment response as well as the role of imaging in patient follow-up and the diagnosis of local tumor recurrence.

Although a small number of patients have other pathologies, the vast majority of bladder cancers are transitional cell carcinomas (TCC), and this chapter will focus solely on this tumor type. The choice of treatment modality in bladder cancer is dependent on many factors; the most important are the stage and histological grade of the tumor, but other important factors include the patient's performance status and co-morbidities, patient preference and the preference and expertise of the treatment center. There are large geographical variations in treatment preferences; in particular, patients with muscle invasive tumors are more likely to be treated with radiotherapy in the UK, compared with the United States.

Imaging following surgery

Transurethral resection and biopsy

Over 80% of bladder cancer patients have superficial (non–muscle invasive) tumors. These patients are usually treated by transurethral resection of the bladder tumor (TURBT). Where there is suspicion of invasion of the bladder muscle wall, deep biopsies into the base of the tumor and into the muscle layer are performed.

Carcinoma of the Bladder, ed. David MacVicar. Published by Cambridge University Press. © Cambridge University Press 2008.

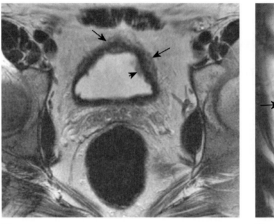
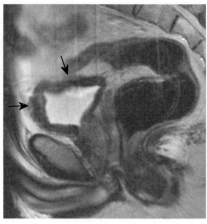

(a)   (b)

Figure 10.1 Post-TURBT appearances of the bladder wall mimicking residual tumor. (a) Transaxial and (b) sagittal T2W images demonstrating abnormal signal intensity of the anterosuperior bladder wall (arrows), with high signal intensity within the muscular layer of the bladder wall and a ragged interface with the extravesical fat. On the left side, in (a), there is intermediate signal intensity mucosal abnormality protruding into the urine (arrowheads). This study was interpreted as showing residual tumor, but on cystectomy the bladder was tumor free and there was extensive post-biopsy inflammatory change present in the dome.

Most patients with superficial bladder tumors do not undergo cross-sectional imaging; however, those patients with suspected muscle invasive disease may be referred for imaging. Cystoscopic biopsy or resection of tumor causes mucosal edema and hemorrhage and localized thinning of the muscle layer. Particularly deep biopsy or resection may cause stranding of the perivesical fat on CT or MRI, owing to inflammation or hemorrhage, or even localized perforation with a perivesical hematoma or collection. These post-operative changes are commonly misinterpreted as residual invasive tumor involving the muscle wall or extending beyond the bladder wall into perivesical fat (Fig. 10.1). Since MRI is particularly sensitive to bladder biopsy effect, it should ideally not be performed for at least four weeks after cystoscopic biopsy or resection, allowing surgical changes to resolve. Where imaging is performed in the immediate post-biopsy period, the radiologist must be aware of this history to avoid overdiagnosis of invasive bladder cancer.

Radical cystectomy

Muscle invasive tumors account for approaching 20% of all bladder cancer cases. In many countries, radical cystectomy is considered the gold standard treatment.

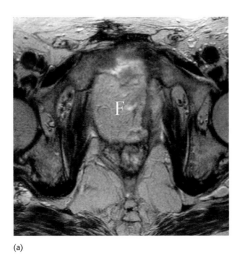
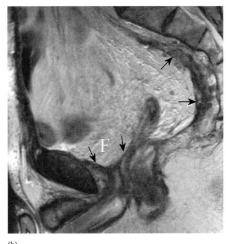

(a)   (b)

Figure 10.2 MR appearances after cystoprostatectomy. (a) Transaxial and (b) sagittal T2W images in a patient who had undergone cystoprostatectomy. In this patient, omental fat (F) fills the bladder bed. The omentum was transposed to stop bowel prolapsing into the bladder bed and thereby preventing it being irradiated should the patient have required radiation therapy after surgery. Note the low-signal fibrotic bands in the bladder bed and irregular low-signal stranding in the presacral space (arrows in (b)) due to the surgery.

Radical (total) cystectomy involves complete excision of the urinary bladder, together with the prostate and seminal vesicles in the male (Fig. 10.2) and hysterectomy, bilateral salpingo-oophrectomy and anterior vaginal wall resection in the female. Urinary drainage must therefore be re-established with either a urinary diversion, usually via an ileal conduit into an abdominal stoma, or a surgically reconstructed bladder (neobladder). Bladder reconstructions are formed from either cecum or small bowel loops which are opened out to form the bladder reservoir. The reconstructed bladder must then be anastomosed to the proximal urethra (orthotopic reconstruction). In some centers, cystectomy with orthotopic bladder reconstruction is performed without prostate and seminal vesicle resection, to preserve sexual function. The incidence of local recurrence in patients undergoing this procedure does not appear to be greater than in those undergoing more radical surgery; however, an unexplained excess in the rate of distant metastases has been observed. Results of more long-term follow-up are awaited [4].

In the early post-operative period, recognized pelvic complications include hematoma or fluid collection, abscess, anastomotic leak and deep venous thrombosis. Simple fluid collections are common; they are typically thin-walled and resolve within a few weeks of surgery. Pelvic hematomas appear of high density on CT in the early phase. Over the first month the contents become gradually iso- or hypodense, as the blood products are resorbed (Fig. 10.3a). On T1-weighted MRI images, subacute and chronic hematomas show a characteristic "concentric ring

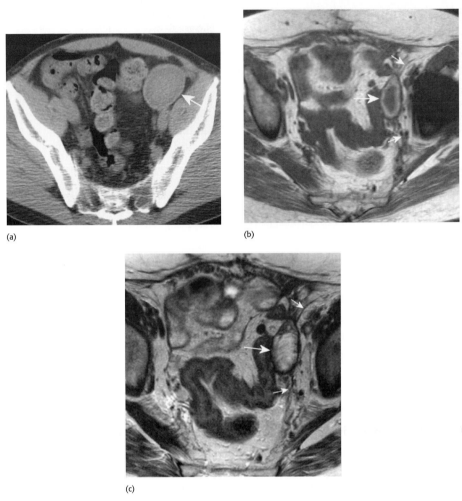

(a)

(b)

(c)

Figure 10.3 Imaging features of pelvic post-surgical hematomas. **(a)** CT image through the pelvis demonstrating a left external iliac hematoma (arrow) within which there is subtle central increased attenuation due to the increased electron density of the retracted clot. Transaxial **(b)** T1W and **(c)** T2W MR images through the pelvis demonstrating a left pelvic sidewall hematoma (long arrow). On the T1W images, there is a characteristic ring appearance with a low signal intensity outer margin (hemosiderin), an inner high signal intensity ring (methemoglobin) and central intermediate signal intensity (deoxyhemoglobin). There is band-like low signal intensity adjacent to the hematoma on the pelvic sidewall (short arrows) which represents post-surgical fibrotic change. Note the midline anterior abdominal wall scar.

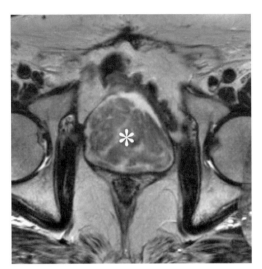

Figure 10.4 MR appearance of Kaltostat hematoma. Transaxial T2W image demonstrating a large mass (*) within the bladder bed after cystoprostatectomy. This demonstrates heterogeneous signal intensity on T2W images with a whorled intermediate signal intensity pattern. The abnormality represents retained unabsorbed Kaltostat, a hemostatic agent, and chronic blood products.

sign"; this appears as central intermediate signal intensity, with a peripheral double ring comprising an inner high signal ring, due to methemoglobin, and a low signal outer ring, due to hemosiderin (Figs. 10.3b and c) [5]. The appearance of chronic pelvic hematomas may be modified by hemostatic gauze (Kaltostat), which has been placed in the surgical bed at the initial operation. These modified hematomas have a mass-like appearance which can be misinterpreted as tumor. The concentric ring sign is absent or barely visible, but they have an unusual central whorled appearance which should be recognized (Fig. 10.4) [6]. Occasionally, surgical sponges or gauze may be retained within the pelvis. If these remain sterile they cause a foreign body reaction and form an aseptic granuloma (gossypiboma). On ultrasound, these are usually hyperechoic with marked posterior shadowing. The CT appearances are variable but are typically of a well-defined hypodense mass, often with an enhancing margin, which may be difficult to distinguish from an abscess. On MRI, the diagnosis can often be made on T2-weighted images, because of a characteristic wavy, folded or sometimes centrally spotted pattern. A radio-opaque strip is variably present, but when seen confirms the diagnosis [7–9].

Orthotopic bladder reconstructions generally have a rounded or oval shape on follow-up CT or MRI, but may be asymmetrical and lobulated. The neobladder wall is thin and appears to consist of a single layer of low signal muscle on T2-weighted MRI images. The bowel folds are commonly effaced on CT, but are more readily seen on MRI protruding into the lumen of the neobladder (Figs. 10.5a and b). Occasionally, an anastomotic leak occurs as an early post-operative complication,

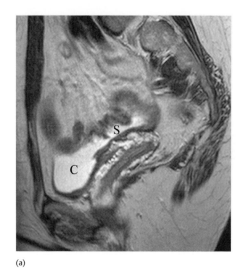
(a)

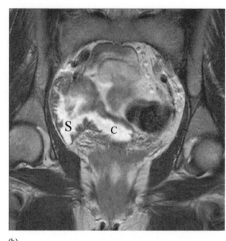
(b)

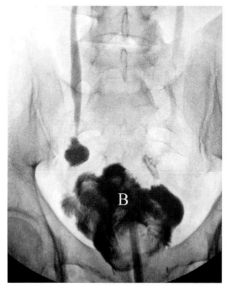
(c)

Figure 10.5 Bladder reconstruction. Sagittal (a) and coronal (b) T2W images showing typical appearances of a bladder orthotopic reconstruction. The urine-filled small bowel (S) and cecum (C) are well seen. (c) Contrast medium study via a Foley catheter with contrast outlining a Hautmann augmentation (B). The contrast medium outlines the small bowel with visualization of the valvulae conniventes. There is retrograde reflux into both ureters.

with the formation of a pelvic urinoma; these may be drained under imaging guidance [10]. A urethral catheter is placed at the time of surgery to protect the urethral anastomosis. It is normal practice to perform a cystogram via the catheter three to four weeks post-operatively to assess for anastomotic leak prior to catheter removal (Fig. 10.5c).

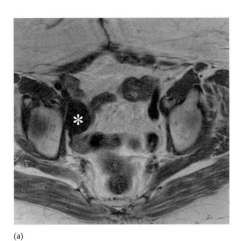 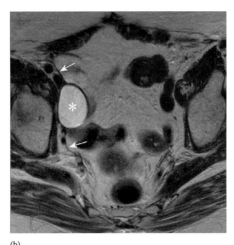

(a)   (b)

Figure 10.6 Right pelvic sidewall lymphocele after cystoprostatectomy. Transaxial (a) T1W and (b) T2W images showing a right-sided unilocular lymphocele (*) directly adjacent to the external iliac vessels. The lymphocele has a thin, well-defined wall and signal intensity equivalent to water. Note the low signal intensity linear change (small arrows in (b)) on the right pelvic sidewall due to the surgical approach.

Bladder cancer surgery usually includes pelvic lymphadenectomy. In these patients, the normal lymphatic drainage from the pelvis and lower limbs is disrupted and pelvic lymphoceles are a relatively common complication. Lymphoceles are recognized by their well-defined smooth margins and thin walls. They usually lie against the pelvic sidewall, and contain clear fluid on ultrasound, CT or MRI (Fig. 10.6). When small, they are often asymptomatic, but larger lymphoceles may cause leg swelling or pain and require image-guided drainage. Recurrence is common and longer-term catheter drainage or sclerotherapy is sometimes required [11].

Intravesical chemotherapy

Repeated bladder instillations of cytotoxic chemotherapy agents, or other agents such as bacille Calmette–Guérin (BCG), are used in recurrent multifocal superficial bladder cancer. These have an irritative effect on the bladder mucosa and may produce severe cystitis with marked thickening and T2-weighted high signal of the bladder wall. A rare complication of intravesical therapy is marked bladder fibrosis and contraction, which may necessitate cystectomy (Fig. 10.7) [12].

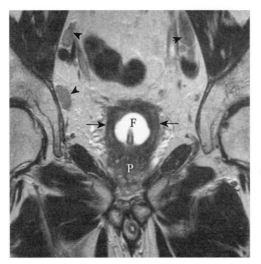

Figure 10.7 Intravesical chemotherapy effect on the bladder. Coronal T2W image in a patient who had undergone multiple courses of intravesical chemotherapy for multifocal superficial bladder tumors. The bladder is of small volume and there is a Foley catheter *in situ* (F). The wall of the bladder (arrows) is irregularly thickened and of low signal intensity. There is a right obturator node and bilateral external iliac nodes (arrowheads) which are of intermediate signal intensity. In these circumstances, it is difficult to know if the lymph nodes are reactive owing to chronic inflammation and fibrosis within the bladder or whether there is early metastatic lymph node disease. The prostate (P) is also of low signal intensity.

Chemotherapy and radiotherapy

Effects on tumor and response evaluation

Systemic chemotherapy and radiotherapy may be used alone or in combination in the treatment of muscle invasive bladder cancer. In clinical practice, response of the tumor is primarily assessed by cystoscopy and biopsy. At our center, patients treated with radiotherapy undergo cystoscopy three months following completion of treatment. CT or MRI is sometimes used to evaluate response, particularly in larger tumors. Imaging evaluation is based upon a subjective assessment of change in tumor volume and the anatomical extent of the mass, as well as intratumoral MR signal intensity changes. Responding tumors show a reduction in size, often with resolution of nodular tumor elements. As response proceeds, any bladder wall disruption regresses and reconstitution occurs with a smooth margin to the wall (Fig. 10.8), although it may become retracted owing to fibrosis. Where there has been complete cystoscopic resection of the intraluminal tumor component prior to chemotherapy or radiotherapy, imaging may only show an area of focal wall thickening. In this situation, a treatment response is represented by a reduction in wall thickening.

Tumor dimensions can be used to provide a more objective assessment of tumor response and are particularly used in clinical trial settings. The commonly used systems are the WHO (World Health Organisation) and RECIST (Response

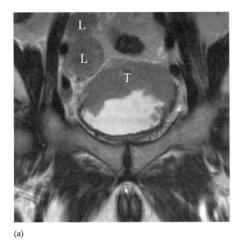
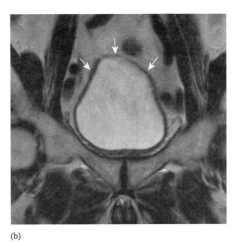

(a)   (b)

Figure 10.8 Excellent response to chemotherapy in bladder cancer. Coronal T2W images (a) pre- and (b) post-chemotherapy. In (a) note the large bladder tumor (T) with substantial right pelvic sidewall lymph node metastases (L). After chemotherapy there has been an excellent response with resolution of the primary bladder tumor and the metastatic nodes. The reconstituted superior bladder wall (arrows) is normal.

Evaluation Criteria in Solid Tumors) criteria, which rely upon bi-dimensional measurements and long-axis measurement, respectively [13,14]. These systems are reasonably effective when applied to uniform rounded masses, but are much less meaningful when used to assess more irregular tumors, or tumors which infiltrate circumferentially around the bladder wall.

On MRI, tumor signal intensity changes are also helpful in evaluating response. Prior to treatment, tumor is typically of intermediate to high signal intensity on T2-weighted images. A treatment response manifests as a reduction in signal intensity, which may be attributed to fibrosis within the tumor. Whereas a reduction in tumor size may occur rapidly, within six to eight weeks of starting treatment, fibrosis may take several months to fully evolve.

Schrier *et al.* [15] have examined the use of dynamic contrast-enhanced MRI in evaluating tumor response to chemotherapy. They found that assessment of early enhancement of the residual bladder mass (occurring within 10 seconds of arterial enhancement) was more accurate than conventional size criteria in determining response after two courses of chemotherapy. Early contrast enhancement is related to tumor neovascularity, and persisting neovascularity after two courses of chemotherapy appears to be a predictor of failure of response to treatment [15,16].

Effects on normal pelvic tissues

Inevitably, normal pelvic tissues will be included within the radiotherapy field and are thus susceptible to radiation damage. Radiation toxicity is because of damage to intracellular DNA, which prevents replication and leads to cell death. Cells that replicate most rapidly, such as epithelial cells, are therefore affected most severely. Early in radiotherapy, cell death occurs and there is tissue necrosis with edema and hemorrhage. Subsequently, vascular damage leads to ischemia, which in the longer term results in tissue fibrosis. Clinically, radiation effects on normal tissues may be divided into acute, in the first three months, subacute, from three months to one year, and chronic, beyond one year. Each of the tissues has a differing sensitivity to radiation damage. The gastrointestinal and urinary tracts are relatively radiosensitive because of their rapid cell turnover. Radiotherapy effects are also dependent upon the radiation dose received, the duration and intensity of radiotherapy, concurrent treatment with chemotherapy (chemoradiation) and patient factors, such as comorbidity with conditions such as hypertension, atherosclerosis and diabetes [17].

Radiation changes within the pelvic tissues may be visible on ultrasound or CT, but are best depicted on MRI. Radiotherapy change of normal bladder is best depicted on thin-section T2-weighted images and in the early stage is manifest as high signal thickening of the bladder mucosa, first affecting the trigone and then other areas. More severe radiation change produces thickening of the bladder wall and high signal within the submucosa and muscle layer (Fig. 10.9) [18]. Typically, with time, the high signal within the bladder wall resolves, although the wall may remain thickened and show low signal because of fibrosis. In some cases, the bladder contracts with a reduction in bladder capacity, leading to severe problems with bladder control. This is most likely to affect patients with pre-existing bladder symptoms. Hemorrhagic cystitis is an uncommon complication which typically occurs in the chronic period following radiotherapy; hemorrhage is owing to telangectasia within the mucosa and bladder wall, which are often visible at cystoscopy. MRI may show intramural hemorrhage, with high signal within the bladder wall on T1-weighted images [19]. Gross radiation damage may result in breakdown of the bladder wall. Initially the wall appears markedly thickened and edematous, and fistulation to the rectum or vagina commonly results. In the long term, strictures of the bladder neck or proximal urethra occasionally occur, although they are more common in patients treated with prostatic or vaginal brachytherapy, when the local radiation dose is higher. The ureters are relatively resistant to

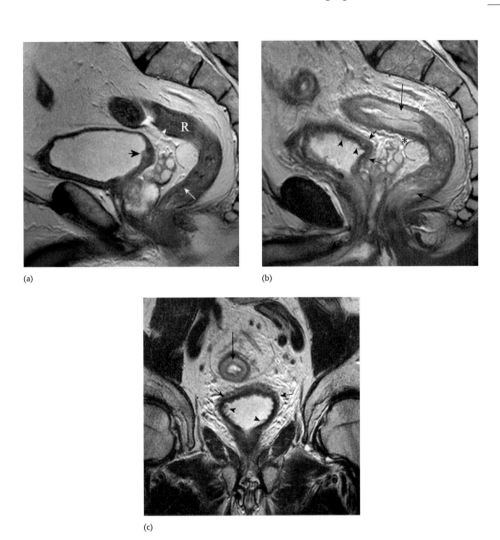

(a)

(b)

(c)

Figure 10.9 Radiation therapy effect. (a) Sagittal T2W image before radiotherapy. Note the small-volume bladder tumor in the posterior wall (arrow). The bladder muscle layer is slightly thickened anteriorly but demonstrates normal signal intensity. The rectum (R) demonstrates low to intermediate signal intensity of the mucosa, submucosa and muscle layer (white arrows). The pelvic fat appears relatively featureless. (b) Sagittal and (c) coronal T2W images post-radiotherapy. The bladder is of reduced volume and there is high signal intensity mucosal edema (arrowheads). The innermost portion of the muscle layer is of low signal intensity but the outer muscle layer and serosa demonstrate intermediate signal (short arrows). The rectosigmoid is now grossly abnormal, with high signal intensity of the mucosa and submucosa (long arrows); there is also increase in signal intensity of the muscle layer (white arrow in (b)). There is increased stranding within the pelvic fat with a small quantity of ascites (asterisk in (b)).

radiation, although radiation-induced strictures do occur in a small number of patients. The most commonly affected site is the distal ureter, just above the vesico-ureteric junction, and strictures are characteristically smooth and tapering.

Radiation effects on the small bowel, sigmoid colon and rectum are common in patients treated with pelvic radiotherapy. While the small bowel is inherently more radiosensitive, radiation change is more common in the distal sigmoid colon and rectum because of their relatively fixed position. Mild changes in the colon and rectum are again best seen on MRI and are manifest as high signal in the submucosa and muscle layer on T2W imaging (Fig. 10.9). In more severe cases, there is marked wall thickening, which is well seen on CT or MRI. Gas may be seen within the bowel wall and ultimately fistulation can occur. In the chronic phase, the bowel wall becomes fibrotic and this may result in strictures which are typically smoothly marginated. Affected segments of small bowel show similar changes, with wall thickening and high signal change in the acute phase (Fig. 10.10) and fibrotic strictures in the chronic phase.

Radiation changes affecting the connective tissues of the pelvis are also visible on CT and MRI. In the acute phase, the pelvic fat and the muscles within the radiation field may show diffuse high signal on T2W MRI images. Thickening of the perirectal fat owing to edema leads to widening of the presacral space. Edema

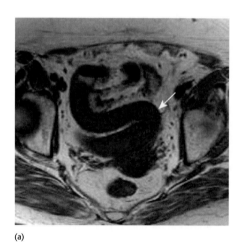
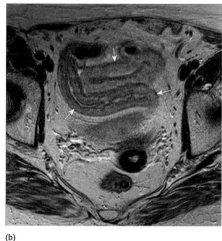

(a)   (b)

Figure 10.10 (a) and (b) small bowel radiation effect after treatment for bladder cancer. Transaxial T1W (a) and T2W (b) images demonstrating grossly abnormal small bowel with multiple thickened loops demonstrating abnormal acute angulation (arrow in (a)) and abnormal high signal intensity throughout the small bowel wall (arrows in (b)).

occurs around the perirectal fascia and is seen as high signal on T2W MRI and as thickening of the fasciae on CT or T1W MRI. In the chronic phase, the perirectal fascia commonly remains thickened owing to fibrosis.

Bone marrow changes occur in virtually all patients treated with radiotherapy. Signal change is commonly seen on MRI in the early phase and is best visualized as high signal intensity on STIR sequences. This occurs within one to two weeks of commencement of treatment and reflects marrow edema and necrosis. Replacement of bone marrow with fat occurs by three to eight weeks after commencement of radiotherapy. On T1W images this is seen as striking high signal intensity, with well-demarcated linear margins corresponding to the radiotherapy field [20].

Radiation-induced insufficiency fractures are common: In a series of patients closely followed up with MRI, these developed in 16 of the 18 patients [21]. Insufficiency fractures occur at the sites of maximum stress because of weight bearing and are commonly bilateral. Most frequently they occur within the sacral alae, parallel to the sacroiliac joints; however, they may also affect the adjacent iliac bones and supra-acetabular regions. Although the fractures may be subclinical, the majority do cause pain, leading to investigation with imaging. On an isotope bone scan, the affected sacrum will show increased tracer uptake, which may be misinterpreted as metastasis, particularly if unilateral. Bilateral fractures may show a characteristic "H" shape pattern of bone scan activity, because of an associated transverse fracture ("Honda sign"), which is more readily recognized. Features on MRI are of low signal on T1W images within the bone adjacent to the sacroiliac joints and of high signal on T2W and STIR images; the signal change is particularly well seen on the STIR sequence. The fracture line cannot be visualized on the T1W images because of low signal within the adjacent bone, but may be seen as a low signal line within the abnormal marrow on the STIR and T2W images (Fig. 10.11). Corresponding CT findings are most commonly of sclerotic bone in the affected area; with thin CT sections, a fracture line, cortical disruption and adjacent callus formation may be seen. Radiologists should be aware of the frequency of this complication to avoid erroneous diagnosis of bone metastases [22]. Metastases may of course occur in these areas, but are usually asymmetrical and may produce cortical destruction and a soft tissue mass.

Radiation osteonecrotic bone is initially sclerotic and is then gradually resorbed and replaced by new bone, a process occurring over several years and known as "creeping substitution." Lytic areas of resorbed bone may occasionally enlarge and simulate a malignant lesion, but absence of periosteal reaction and soft tissue mass

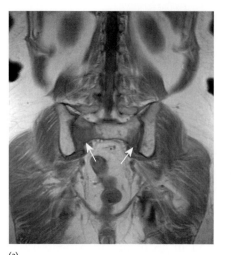 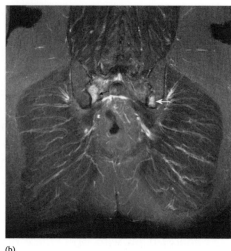

(a)   (b)

Figure 10.11 Sacral insufficiency fractures after radiotherapy for bladder cancer. Coronal T1W (a) and STIR (b) images demonstrating abnormal intermediate signal intensity in the lateral aspects of the sacrum bilaterally (arrows in (a)), with high signal intensity present at the same sites on the STIR sequence. However, a fracture line (black arrow in (b)) is visible within the right sacral wing on the STIR image. An additional area of high signal intensity on the STIR sequence is noted in the medial left ileum (white arrow), which is less obvious on the T1W image but represents a further site of marrow edema owing to altered stresses.

are reassuring signs. Not infrequently, infection will coexist with radiation osteo-necrosis. This leads to bone destruction with a soft tissue mass and often a pathological fracture. In the pelvis, the pubic bones are most commonly affected. Differentiation from bone metastasis on imaging is often impossible, but occasionally gas is seen within the mass or there is an adjacent pelvic abscess which indicates infection. Affected patients often have a history of severe radiation bowel or bladder disease requiring surgery [23].

Avascular necrosis (AVN) occurs most commonly in oncology patients treated with chemotherapy and steroids, but is also related to radiotherapy. The femoral heads are most frequently affected. MRI is the modality of choice for the early detection of AVN; the characteristic appearance is the "double-line sign" which is seen on T2-weighted images as an outer low signal line, representing necrosis, and an inner high signal line, representing hyperemia and inflammation [24].

Skeletal muscle within the radiotherapy field may develop radiotherapy change. This may occur within three weeks of the onset of radiotherapy and is initially manifest as homogenous high signal within the muscle on T2-weighted images (Fig. 10.12). In the long term, atrophy and fibrosis may develop.

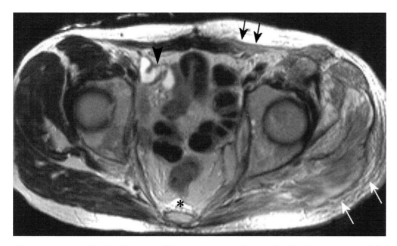

Figure 10.12 Radiation therapy effect on the muscles and soft tissue. Transaxial T2W image of a bladder cancer patient who had been treated by cystoprostatectomy and then had radiotherapy to the left pelvis for an inguinal recurrence. Note the difference in signal intensity between the muscles in the right pelvis and the left, there being abnormal high signal intensity on the left side. This is also evident in the rectus abdominis muscles, where the lateral portion of the left rectus abdominis muscle is of high signal intensity (black arrows) compared to the normal right side. There has been an increase in edema and stranding within the subcutaneous fat (small white arrows). A small amount of presacral fluid (asterisk) is noted. The patient's ileal loop is seen in the right anterior pelvis (arrowhead).

Evaluation of residual masses following treatment

Following treatment with chemotherapy and/or radiotherapy, a bladder tumor may resolve completely. However, with muscle invasive tumors there is commonly a residual abnormality, which may be a bladder wall nodule or mass or a focal or diffuse area of bladder wall thickening. These lesions present a diagnostic dilemma for the clinician, who needs to know whether there is active tumor within this residual mass, since patients in whom residual tumor is identified may be suitable for salvage surgery. For this reason, radiotherapy patients are evaluated with cystoscopy and biopsy at the end of treatment. Cystoscopic assessment is confined to the inner surface of the bladder but cross-sectional imaging is able to give additional information about the outer bladder wall, the perivesical tissues and the pelvic nodes. MRI is superior to CT in the assessment of residual bladder abnormalities, in that high-resolution T2W images can identify the individual layers of the bladder wall, can better depict the margins of the residual mass and the signal intensity of the mass can be scrutinized. Active tumor is more likely to show intermediate to high signal, whereas fibrosis is typically of low signal on T2W images.

Dynamic contrast-enhanced MRI

There has been a variety of studies looking at the use of dynamic contrast-enhanced MRI in the investigation of treated bladder cancer patients to assist in the differentiation between tumor, edema and fibrosis. Over the last 15 years, these techniques have developed together with the evolution of faster MR scanners. The original studies were limited to assessing enhancement of a region of interest on a single slice. However, the current generation of MRI equipment allows assessment of dynamic data for a volume which includes the majority of the bladder. In one of the early studies, Barentsz *et al.* [25] studied a group of 61 bladder cancer patients one to four weeks following transurethral resection or biopsy. They used a single-slice turbo FLASH (fast low-angle shot) sequence to acquire images every 1.25 seconds and used a threshold of 10 seconds from the beginning of arterial enhancement to distinguish tumor from fibrosis, with tumor enhancing more rapidly than benign tissue. The accuracy of diagnosis was improved from 79% for non-enhanced images to 90% with the dynamic contrast-enhanced technique.

Dobson *et al.* [26] also used a single-slice technique, with images acquired every 8 seconds to compare dynamic enhancement profiles for bladder tumor and non-tumor. They found that an enhancement ratio of greater than 1.54 over baseline at 80 seconds post-contrast injection was discriminatory for tumor. This technique had a high sensitivity and negative predictive value, but a low specificity and positive predictive value for detection of tumor. Negative predictive values were 100 and 93% at 4 and 12 months post-radiotherapy respectively, i.e. a negative result was highly predictive of absence of tumor [26]. Dynamic contrast enhanced (DCE) MRI has also been used to assess response of bladder cancer to chemotherapy, as described in the earlier section.

In our institution, the DCE MRI protocol on a 1.5T system includes high-resolution T2-weighted images for localization of the bladder lesion. The dynamic series are acquired using a rapid 3D T1-weighted gradient echo sequence (VIBE), with parallel imaging resulting in a volume being acquired every 2.6 seconds. The acquired volume has a craniocaudal extent of 8 cm, which is sufficient to cover the majority of the bladder. An infusion pump is used to inject a dose of 0.1 mMol/kg gadolinium-DTPA and imaging of the tissue volume continues for three minutes post-injection. Curves of enhancement against time are obtained for selected regions of interest. In line with previous experience, our results have shown differences in enhancement curve shapes between tumor and fibrosis; tumor enhances rapidly and then plateaus, while fibrosis shows a more gradual uptake until the curves eventually overlap (Figs. 10.13–10.15). These differences in enhancement curve shape can also be shown by calculation of the area under the concentration–time curve (AUC) at 60 and 90 seconds with AUC values being significantly higher in tumor. Our results also concur with Dobson *et al.* [26] who found that increased relative signal intensity (rSI) at 80 seconds post-arterial enhancement was predictive of tumor.

Patterns of tumor recurrence

The expected pattern of tumor recurrence is dependent upon the initial treatment modality. Patients who have undergone radical cystectomy are most likely to develop bladder bed recurrence, and pelvic lymph node and distant metastases (most commonly to liver, lung and bone). The median time to recurrence post-cystectomy is 8–18 months, with most recurrences occurring within two years [27,28]. Recurrence is more likely in non–organ-confined tumors (T3 and T4) and in those with metastases in pelvic nodes. These patients also recur more quickly, with a median time to recurrence of 12 months [29,30]. Local recurrence accounts for approximately 10–30% of all recurrences and commonly presents with lower pelvic or perineal pain, lower limb or genital edema and sometimes priapism (Figs. 10.16a–d) [27,28,30,31]. Up to 50% of patients with local recurrence also have distant metastases [27]. Surgical cases also have an appreciable risk of urethral recurrence. The frequency of this varies considerably between series, from less than 1% to over 10% of patients, and is dependent upon a number of risk factors, the most important of which is involvement of the prostate with tumor [27,28,32]. In certain high-risk patients, the urethra is prophylactically resected at the time of cystoprostatectomy. The risk of urethral recurrence appears to be lower in patients who have undergone orthotopic bladder reconstruction as opposed to those with urinary diversions. This may be owing to selection bias, but it has also been postulated that continued urine flow through the urethra may have a protective effect [33].

Following radiotherapy, over 90% of tumor recurrences occur locally within the bladder [34]. In these patients, early detection of recurrence is important as it may allow salvage surgery. MRI is superior to CT in the detection of local bladder

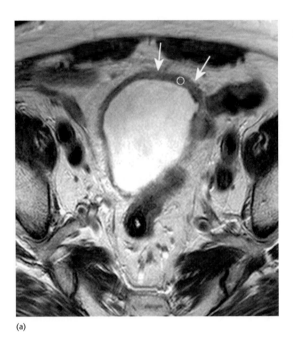

(a)

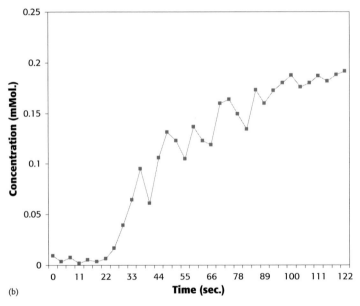

(b)

Figure 10.13 Dynamic contrast-enhanced MRI demonstrating fibrosis. (a) Transaxial T2W image of a bladder cancer patient treated with chemoradiotherapy two years previously. There is bladder wall thickening and stranding extending into the perivesical fat anterolaterally on the left (arrows). (b) Enhancement curve from a region of interest marked over the area of thickening (circle in (a)). Initial enhancement is later than 22 seconds with a slow and gradual increase in concentration of contrast. These appearances are typical for fibrosis. This was confirmed at biopsy.

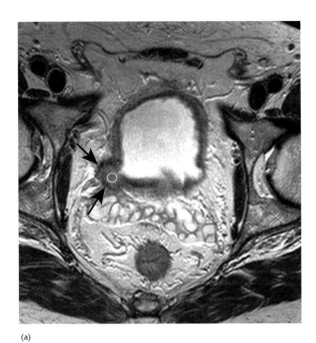

(a)

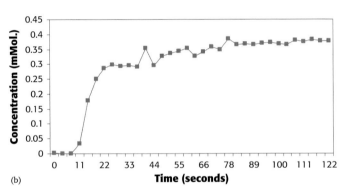

(b)

Figure 10.14 Dynamic contrast-enhanced MRI demonstrating tumor. (a) Transaxial T2W image demonstrating soft tissue thickening at the right vesico-ureteric junction (arrow) in this patient who had been treated with neoadjuvant chemotherapy for a bladder tumor. (b) Enhancement curve from a region of interest over the right vesico-ureteric junction (circle in (a)) in the same patient demonstrates early and rapid enhancement, which is the typical enhancement profile of tumor.

recurrence. The typical appearance of recurrent tumor on T2-weighted images is of an intermediate to high signal nodule, most often involving the mucosal surface, but frequently also within the bladder muscle layer. Recurrence may occur at any site within the treated bladder, but most frequently in the area of the primary tumor. Recurrence is also likely to occur at the margins of the radiotherapy field,

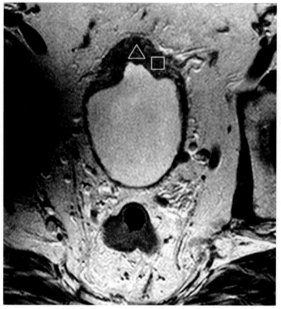

(a)

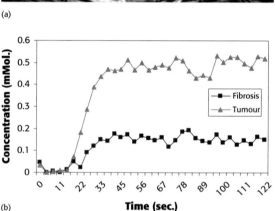

(b)

Figure 10.15 Dynamic contrast-enhanced MRI demonstrating fibrosis and tumor. (a) Transaxial T2W image of a bladder cancer patient treated with neoadjuvant chemotherapy. There is marked thickening of the anterior bladder wall, which appears of uniform intermediate signal intensity. Regions of interest for enhancement curves have been selected in the midline (△) and to the left (□). (b) Enhancement curve for the midline area of abnormality (△) shows rapid and intense enhancement consistent with residual tumor. The enhancement curve more laterally (□) within the anterior bladder wall shows a more gradual and delayed enhancement with a smaller area under the curve relative to the tumor. The bladder wall therefore shows two distinct enhancement profiles consistent with central tumor and peripheral fibrosis, which were indistinguishable on the T2W image.

particularly along the pelvic floor and around the distal ureters or ureteric orifices, when hydronephrosis is a common presenting sign.

Patients with bladder TCC are at increased risk of developing TCC elsewhere within the urinary tract. The risk of upper tract carcinoma can be stratified according to various risk factors; patients with a solitary, low grade, superficial tumor have a risk of 1% or less, whereas patients with carcinoma *in situ*, high grade superficial tumors, failure of primary treatment or distal ureteric involvement have a risk of 10% or more. Most new upper tract tumors occur between two and four years after initial treatment [35].

Pelvic sidewall lymph nodes are a common site of metastases. In patients previously treated with radiotherapy, nodal metastases usually occur concurrently with bladder recurrence, solitary nodal recurrence occurring in approximately 10% of cases [36]. As in primary staging, diagnosis of nodal metastases on cross-sectional imaging is largely based on size, with CT and MRI having broadly equivalent accuracies. However, heterogeneous nodal signal, similar to that of tumor, and central necrosis are additional signs of malignancy on MRI (Fig. 10.16e). Pelvic lymphadenopathy generally precludes the possibility of curative salvage surgery, although it should be remembered that enlarged nodes may occasionally be reactive rather than metastatic. MRI with ultrasmall superparamagnetic iron oxide particles (ferumoxtran-10) has been shown to improve the detection of nodal metastases in the initial staging of bladder cancer [37], but its use has not been assessed in the context of tumor recurrence.

FDG-PET scanning is of little value in the assessment of local disease recurrence for bladder cancer, because renal excretion of the radio-isotope produces massive urinary hyperintensity which masks any tumor activity. There is, however, a possible role for FDG-PET in the assessment of lymph node and more distant metastases. It is currently not used in routine clinical practice in the follow-up of bladder cancer. Other isotopes which do not accumulate in the bladder may be of value in the future; preliminary results on the use of ^{11}C-choline in the staging of bladder cancer have been promising [38].

Follow-up of treated bladder cancer

There is surprisingly little literature regarding the radiological follow-up of treated bladder cancer. The rationale for follow-up of any cancer is that early detection of recurrence may allow more successful second-line treatment – this is most important when early diagnosis can lead to curative surgery. Imaging plays little part in the follow-up of patients with superficial bladder cancers, in whom follow-up is by clinical evaluation, cystoscopy and urine cytology.

Cystoscopy is also the mainstay of follow-up in patients with muscle invasive tumors undergoing bladder preserving treatment (radiotherapy, chemoradiotherapy or partial cystectomy). At our center, cystoscopy is performed four-monthly up to 12 months, then six-monthly up to two years, and then annually. The additional value of CT or MRI in the follow-up of these patients is contentious, with no literature to support its routine use. An ongoing multicenter UK trial of chemo-radiotherapy includes close MRI follow-up of patients and it is hoped this will provide evidence of its value. Patients who develop recurrent tumor should undergo

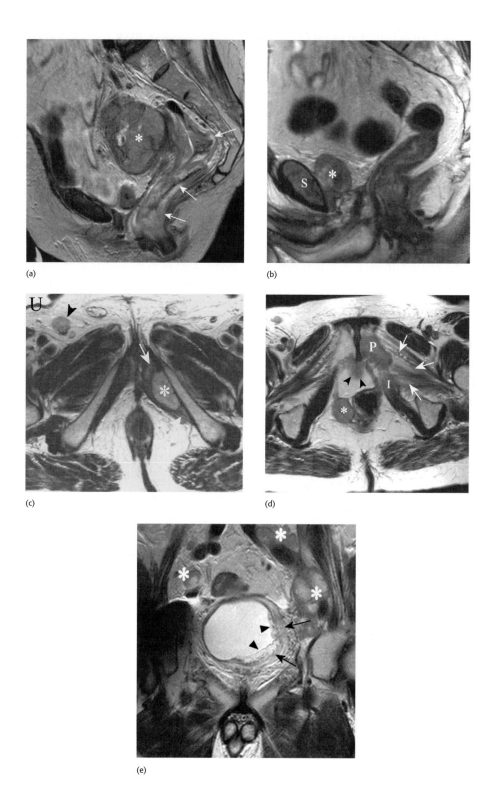

(a)

(b)

(c)

(d)

(e)

restaging with CT or MRI (MRI being more accurate) to determine whether salvage cystectomy is possible.

Imaging follow-up after cystectomy is also a contentious issue. In the UK, the majority of patients are followed up with excretory urography and radionuclide renography, with the use of cross-sectional imaging in appropriate cases. The main aims of this approach are to monitor drainage of the urinary tract, so that obstruction can be promptly diagnosed and treated, and to monitor the upper tracts for tumor. The intensity of upper-tract follow-up is dependent upon risk stratification. High-risk patients are typically followed up with annual IVU or contrast loopogram. CT urography should be considered in high-risk groups because of its increased sensitivity [39]. CT is a sensitive modality for the detection of local recurrence and distant metastases and is preferred to MRI. The large majority of patients with recurrence after cystectomy have incurable disease. Although chemotherapy can provide good palliation, there is no evidence that early detection of relapse improves outcome [40]. It can be argued that more intensive follow-up should be directed at patients with T3 and T4 tumors and those with positive nodes at surgery, as they have the highest risk of recurrence. In this case, follow-up should be concentrated within the first 18 months after treatment, when the incidence of recurrence is greatest [41].

Given the lack of evidence of survival benefit from intensive follow-up, it is unsurprising that no clear guidance for its use exists. The Royal College of Radiologists recommends CT as the modality of choice for follow-up after cystectomy, but

---

Caption for Figure 10.16 Bladder cancer recurrence. (a) Sagittal T2W image in a patient who had a previous cystectomy demonstrating a predominantly solid high signal intensity central pelvic tumor recurrence (*). Note the abnormal high signal intensity within the rectum and anal canal (long arrows) owing to radiation therapy effect. (b) Sagittal T2W image in a patient who had undergone cystoprostatectomy demonstrating a bladder bed recurrence (*). This mass is adherent to the symphysis pubis (S). (c) Transaxial T2W image demonstrating a left pelvic recurrence (*) involving the ischiocavernosus, which demonstrates increased signal intensity (arrows). A right inguinal metastatic lymph node (arrowheads) is also noted. Note the right iliac fossa stoma bag containing urine (U). (d) Transaxial T2W image showing multifocal pelvic recurrent tumor post cystoprostatectomy with masses seen involving the right puborectalis component of the levator ani muscle (*), the left pubic bone (P) and the retropubic bladder base (arrowheads). Note the increased signal intensity in the anterioinferior portion of the left obturator internus muscle (I) as well as obturator externus and pectoneus muscles (arrows). The muscle findings are an edematous reaction to the presence of the symphysis pubis tumor which has extended out into the obturator foramen. (e) Coronal T2W image showing bilateral pelvic metastastic lymph nodes (*) in a bladder cancer patient treated with chemotherapy and radiotherapy. The lymph nodes show heterogenous signal intensity with central necrosis. The left bladder wall shows marked mucosal edema (arrowheads) and wall thickening with high signal intensity (arrows) secondary to radiotherapy. The reason for the unilateral bladder change is unclear as the whole bladder was included in the radiotherapy field.

does not advise on follow-up intervals [42]. The European Urological Society recommends a combination of chest radiography, abdominal ultrasound every four months following cystectomy, and CT for node positive patients, but does not advise on the duration of follow-up [43]. Recommended post-cystectomy follow-up regimes in North America are generally more intensive, with abdominal and pelvic CT or MRI typically performed at three months, then six-monthly up to two years, and then annually up to five years [27,40].

Summary

Bladder cancer is currently treated by surgery, radiotherapy or chemoradiotherapy, and these treatment modalities induce imaging changes in the pelvis which should be recognized by radiologists. Surgical effects include normal post-cystectomy and orthotopic bladder reconstruction appearances as well as pelvic post-operative complications. Radiotherapy induces changes within the tumor, but also within normal pelvic tissues, and these are best depicted using MRI. After radiotherapy, any residual bladder mass is a diagnostic challenge and dynamic contrast-enhanced MRI is superior to non-contrast MRI in distinguishing residual tumor from post-treatment fibrosis. Response to radiotherapy is currently assessed using a combination of cystoscopy and imaging, but dynamic contrast-enhanced MRI shows promise in the early prediction of treatment response. Follow-up protocols after treatment for bladder cancer vary widely and there is no clear evidence that these are beneficial in terms of patient outcome.

ACKNOWLEDGEMENT

The authors are grateful to Stephanie Donaldson, North Western Medical Physics, Christie Hospital, Manchester, for data and images on dynamic contrast-enhanced MRI.

REFERENCES

1. Husband J E, Olliff J F, Williams M P *et al.* Bladder cancer: staging with CT and MR imaging. *Radiology* 1989; **173**: 435–40.
2. Kim B, Semelka R C, Ascher S M *et al.* Bladder tumour staging: comparison of contrast-enhanced CT, T1- and T2-weighted MR imaging, dynamic gadolinium-enhanced imaging and late gadolinium-enhanced imaging. *Radiology* 1994; **193**: 239–45.

3. Tanimoto A, Yuasa Y, Imai Y *et al.* Bladder tumour staging: comparison of conventional and gadolinium-enhanced dynamic MR imaging and CT. *Radiology* 1992; **185**: 741–7.

4. Hautmann R E, Stein J P. Neobladder with prostatic capsule and seminal-sparing cystectomy for bladder cancer: a step in the wrong direction. *Urol Clin North Am.* 2005; **32**: 177–85.

5. Hahn P F, Saini S, Stark D D *et al.* Intraabdominal hematoma: the concentric-ring sign in MR imaging. *AJR Am J Roentgenol* 1987; **148**: 115–19.

6. Naik K S, Carrington B M, Yates W, Clarke N W. The post-cystectomy pseudotumour sign: MRI appearances of a modified chronic pelvic haematoma due to retained haemostatic gauze. *Clin Radiol* 2000; **55**: 970–4.

7. Kokubo T, Itai Y, Ohtomo K *et al.* Retained surgical sponges: CT and US appearance. *Radiology* 1987; **165**: 415–18.

8. Kalovidouris A, Kehagias D, Moulopoulos L *et al.* Abdominal retained surgical sponges: CT appearance. *Eur Radiol* 1999; **9**: 1407–10.

9. Sugimura H, Tamura S, Kakitsubata Y *et al.* Magnetic resonance imaging of retained surgical sponges. Case report. *Clin Imaging* 1992; **16**: 259–62.

10. Heaney M D, Francis I R, Cohan R H *et al.* Orthotopic neobladder reconstruction: findings on excretory urography and CT. *AJR Am J Roentgenol* 1999; **172**: 1213–20.

11. vanSonnenberg E, Wittich G R, Casola G *et al.* Lymphoceles: imaging characteristics and percutaneous management. *Radiology* 1986; **161**: 593–6.

12. Nieder A M, Sved P D, Stein J P *et al.* Cystoprostatectomy and orthotopic ileal neobladder reconstruction for management of bacille Calmette Guerin-induced bladder contractures. *Urology.* 2005; **65**: 909–12.

13. Miller A B, Hoogstraten B, Staquet M, Winkler A. Reporting results of cancer treatment. *Cancer* 1981; **47**: 207–14.

14. Therasse P, Arbuck S G, Eisenhauer E A *et al.* New guidelines to evaluate the response to treatment in solid tumours. *J Natl Cancer Inst* 2000; **92**: 205–16.

15. Schrier B P, Peters M, Barentsz J O, Witjes J A. Evaluation of chemotherapy with magnetic resonance imaging in patients with regionally metastatic or unresectable bladder cancer. *Eur Urol* 2006; **49**: 698–703.

16. Barentsz J O, Berger-Hartog O, Witjes J A *et al.* Evaluation of chemotherapy in advanced urinary bladder cancer with fast dynamic contrast-enhanced MR imaging. *Radiology* 1998; **207**: 791–7.

17. Johnson R J, Carrington B M. Pelvic radiation disease. *Clin Radiol* 1992; **45**: 4–12.

18. Sugimura K, Carrington B M, Quivey J M, Hricak H. Postirradiation changes in the pelvis: assessment with MR imaging. *Radiology* 1990; **175**: 805–13.

19. Worawattanakul S, Semelka R C, Kelekis N L. Post radiation hemorrhagic cystitis: MR findings. *Magn Reson Imaging* 1997; **15**: 1103–6.

20. Blomlie V, Rofstad E K, Skjonsberg A *et al.* Female pelvic bone marrow: serial MR imaging before, during and after radiation therapy. *Radiology* 1995; **194**: 537–43.

21. Blomlie V, Rofstad E K, Talle K *et al.* Incidence of radiation-induced insufficiency fractures of the female pelvis: evaluation with MR imaging. *AJR Am J Roentgenol* 1996; **167**: 1205–10.

22. Kanberoglu K, Mihmanli I, Kurugoglu S *et al.* Bone marrow changes adjacent to the sacroiliac joints after pelvic radiotherapy mimicking metastases on MRI. *Eur Radiol* 2001; **11**: 1748–52.

23. Wignall T A, Carrington B M, Logue J P. Post-radiotherapy osteomyelitis of the symphysis pubis: computed tomographic features. *Clin Radiol* 1998; **53**: 126–30.

24. Mitchell D G, Rao V M, Dalinka M K *et al.* Femoral head avascular necrosis: correlation of MR imaging, radiographic staging, radionuclide imaging, and clinical findings. *Radiology* 1987; **162**: 709–15.

25. Barentsz J O, Jager G J, van Vierzen P B *et al.* Staging urinary bladder cancer after transurethral biopsy: value of fast dynamic contrast-enhanced MR imaging. *Radiology* 1996; **201**: 185–93.

26. Dobson M J, Carrington B M, Collins C D *et al.* The assessment of irradiated bladder carcinoma using dynamic contrast-enhanced MR imaging. *Clin Radiol* 2001; **56**: 94–8.

27. Bochner B H, Montie J E, Lee C T. Follow-up strategies and management of recurrence in urologic oncology bladder cancer: Invasive bladder cancer. *Urol Clin North Am*; 2003; **30**: 777–89.

28. Malkowicz S B, van Poppel H, Mickisch G *et al.* Muscle-invasive urothelial carcinoma of the bladder. *Urology* 2007; **69**(1 suppl): 3–16.

29. Stein J P, Lieskovsky G, Cote R *et al.* Radical cystectomy in the treatment of invasive bladder cancer: long-term results in 1,054 patients. *J Clin Oncol* 2001; **19**: 666–75.

30. Koh D M, Husband J E. Patterns of recurrence of bladder carcinoma following radical cystectomy. *Cancer Imaging* 2003; **3**: 96–100.

31. Hassan J M, Cookson M S, Smith J A Jr., Chang S S. Patterns of initial transitional cell recurrence in patients after cystectomy. *J Urol* 2006; **175**: 2054–7.

32. Hassan J M, Cookson M S, Smith J A Jr., Chang S S. Urethral recurrence in patients following orthotopic urinary diversion. *J Urol* 2004; **172**(4 Pt 1): 1338–41.

33. Nieder A M, Sved P D, Gomez P *et al.* Urethral recurrence after cystoprostatectomy: implications for urinary diversion and monitoring. *Urology* 2004; **64**: 950–4.

34. Van der Werf-Messing B, Menon R S, Hop W C. Cancer of the urinary bladder category T2, T3 (NxM0) treated by interstitial radium implant: second report. *Int J Radiat Oncol Biol Phys* 1983; **9**: 481–5.

35. Kenworthy P, Tanguay S, Dinney C P. The risk of upper tract recurrence following cystectomy in patients with transitional cell carcinoma involving the distal ureter. *J Urol* 1996; **155**(February): 501–3.

36. Cowan R A, McBain C A, Ryder W D *et al.* Radiotherapy for muscle invasive carcinoma of the bladder: results of a randomized trial comparing conventional whole bladder with dose-escalated partial bladder radiotherapy. *Int J Radiat Oncol Biol Phys* 2004; **59**: 197–207.

37. Deserno W M, Harisinghani M G, Taupitz M *et al.* Urinary bladder cancer: preoperative nodal staging with ferumoxtran-10-enhanced MR imaging. *Radiology* 2004; **233**(2): 449–56.

38. Picchio M, Treiber U, Beer A J *et al*. Value of 11C-choline PET and contrast-enhanced CT for staging of bladder cancer: correlation with histopathologic findings. *J Nucl Med* 2006; **47**: 938–44.

39. Browne R F, Meehan C P, Colville J *et al*. Transitional cell carcinoma of the upper urinary tract: spectrum of imaging findings. *Radiographics* 2005; **25**: 1609–27.

40. Westney O L, Pisters L L, Pettaway C A *et al*. Presentation, methods of diagnosis and therapy for pelvic recurrence following radical cystectomy for transitional cell carcinoma of the bladder. *J Urol* 1998; **159**: 792–5.

41. Slaton J W, Swanson D A, Grossman H B, Dinney C P. A stage specific approach to tumour surveillance after radical cystectomy for transitional cell carcinoma of the bladder. *J Urol* 1999; **162**: 710–14.

42. Recommendations for Cross-Sectional Imaging in Cancer Management: Computed tomography – CT, Magnetic resonance imaging – MRI, Positron emission tomography – PET, Issue 2. The Royal College of Radiologists (2006), London, UK. RCR Ref No RCR (06)1.

43. European Association of Urology. *Guidelines*, Arnhem, The Netherlands: European Association of Urology, 2006.

Index

accelerated M-VAC chemotherapy, 130–131
  see also CMV chemotherapy; gemcitabine/cisplatin
    (GC) chemotherapy; M-VAC chemotherapy
adenocarcinoma
  imaging, 42–43
  non-urachal, 43
  pathology, 17–18
  urachal, 18, 43
  see also small cell (neuroendocrine) carcinoma;
    squamous cell carcinoma (SCC)
adjuvant chemotherapy, 125, 129
  see also neoadjuvant chemotherapy
adriamycin (methotrexate, vinblastine, adriamycin,
    cisplatin) *see* M-VAC chemotherapy
air-insufflation technique, 57
anastomosis
  Bricker, 101
  uretero-intestinal, 100
  Wallace, 101
Aristolochia fangchi, 24
avascular necrosis (AVN), 160

Bacille Calmette–Guérin (BCG), 28–29
benign papilloma, 12
benign tumors, 19
biopsy, transurethral resection, 147–148
bladder cancer
  chemotherapy for, 125–133
  clinical features
    anatomical predisposition, 24
    chemical aspects, 24
    clinical presentation and initial management, 26–27
    environmental aspects, 24
    epidemiology, 23
    etiology, 24–25
    genetic predisposition, 25
    staging and grading effects, 27–29
  cystoscopy for, *see* cystoscopy
  follow-up, 137–143
  imaging
    characteristics of histological subtypes, 41–48
    clinical presentation and management, 31–32

    diagnostic evaluation, 32–41
    hematuria, 31
  management in UK, 25–26
  pathology, 1–21
    adenocarcinoma, 17–18
    benign and low malignant potential urothelial
      lesions, 12
    benign tumors, 19
    cancer type features, 5
    diffuse or multifocal tumor, 5
    etiology, 4
    genetics and multifocality, 4
    grading aspects, 5
    histopathological approach, 4–12
    inverted papilloma, 12
    lymphovascular (LVSI) space invasion
      aspects, 5
    metastatic cancer, 19
    PUNLMP, 12
    rare cancers, 19
    renal pelvis and ureter, 19–20
    small cell (neuroendocrine) carcinoma, 18–19
    squamous cell carcinoma (SCC), 15–17
    staging aspects, 5
    TNM pathological staging, 5–8
    urethral carcinomas, 20–21
    urinary cytology aspects, 21
    urothelial carcinoma and, 12–15
    urothelial papilloma, 12
  radiological staging, 51–74
  surgery for, 93–103
    cystectomy, 94–100
    pelvic lymphadenectomy, 99
    urethrectomy, 97–98
    urinary diversion aspects, 100–103
  TNM staging, 52
  transurethral resection evaluation, 93
  urothelial tumors, 2–3
  WHO classification of urothelial tumors, 1–2
  see also muscle invasive bladder cancer; superficial
    bladder cancer; urothelial carcinomas
blue-light cystoscopy, 27